PLAGUE DOCTORS

PLAGUE DOCTORS

HOW HAWAI'I BATTLED THE PANDEMIC

JONATHAN DWORKIN, MD

WATERMARK
PUBLISHING

ISBN 978-1-948011-66-2

Cover photography istock/daikokuebisu, istock/Arand;
interior photography Jonathan Dworkin used with permission

Library of Congress Control Number: 2021946311

Design and production
Kristin Kaleinani Lipman

Watermark Publishing
1000 Bishop St., Ste. 806
Honolulu, HI 96813
Telephone 1-808-587-7766
Toll-free 1-866-900-BOOK
sales@bookshawaii.net
www.bookshawaii.net

10 9 8 7 6 5 4 3 2 1

Printed in Korea

For Barry Dworkin, who never had a boss

Fear of gods or law of man there was none to restrain them. As for the first, they judged it to be the same whether they worshiped them or not, as they saw all alike perishing; and for the last, no one expected to live to be brought to trial for his offenses, but each felt that a far severer sentence had already been passed upon them all and hung over their heads.

—THUCYDIDES ON THE PLAGUE OF ATHENS

CONTENTS

ACKNOWLEDGMENTS

This book is an account of the first year of the COVID-19 pandemic from my perspective as an infectious diseases doctor in Hawai'i. It covers the confusion that gripped the hospitals in the early days, the response that followed, and the eventual resolution that led the state out of the crisis. I discuss the medical challenges in managing the disease, alternating between those problems and the broader pandemic response, which I assisted in Hawai'i.

In telling the tale, at times I zoom out to the global scale, then refocus on the particular dynamics playing out in the Islands. I include at the end of the chapters a brief section titled "Backstory," which is a series of Facebook posts I wrote during the height of the crisis. This may be of interest to readers who want to delve further into details of the arguments over the pandemic, or better understand my thinking as it evolved in real time. The themes that emerge are what the pandemic revealed about society, and the relationship between human behavior and disease.

There are a lot of people whose assistance made this book possible. Within the Queen's division of infectious diseases, I am indebted to Joe Koo and Royden Young for both support and counsel. I would also like to thank James Joyner, Heath Chung, Larry Day, and Erlaine Bello for useful conversations. In the pulmonary and critical care division, I derived benefit from speaking with Scott Gallagher, Chris Fiack, Bret Tatsuno, Russell Gilbert, Jordan Lee, Reid Ikeda, Gehan Davendra, and Stephanie Guo. In the internal medicine division, I would like to thank Masayuki Nogi, Ryan Honda, Malia Ramirez, Kuo Lian, Lester Morehead, Christina Chong, Karen Dang, Grant Chen, Matt Brown, Ynhu Le, Rob Eager, John Misailidis, Judy Rudnick, Amanda Haley, Sandra Loo, and Ali Chisti. Lynell Newmarch provided me with early clinical information. My former stewardship colleague, Lynn Matsukawa, was also a source of information, as was the head of the Queen's pharmacy, Marcy Rapp.

There were many people at the University of Hawai'i John A. Burns School of Medicine, as well as the Queen's clinical trials group, who helped on research questions during the pandemic. Todd Seto and

Dominic Chow, as well as May Vawer, helped with drug and clinical trial issues. Tim Brown provided expertise in modeling, as did Lee Altenberg, Tom Ramsey, and DeWolfe Miller. Sumner La Croix provided me with relevant information and analysis on Hawai'i's economy. Lee Buenconsejo, Al Katz, Robert Perkinson, S. Y. Tan, Joel Brown, and Bruce Soll each pushed me in helpful directions at critical phases.

Colleagues and mentors from Brown University also assisted me, mostly in the form of deep dives on particular questions. This includes Leonard Mermel, Ben Westley, and Josh Fischer.

Colleagues in the Kurdish region, in particular Hawar Mykhan and Rebeen Saeed, helped me understand the outbreak globally.

On the Big Island, I would like to thank James Madison, Crystal Hammer, and Britney Spivak for being excellent colleagues in managing COVID-19 patients in our rural setting. I've also benefited from conversations about the epidemic on this island with Alex DiTullio, Terence Jones, Stafford Clarry, Elizabeth Bush, Miles Matsumara, William Showalter, Kaohimanu Akiona, Nikki Switzer, Buzz Hollander, John Kurap, Melissa Pulling, Ali Bairos, John Dawson, Chery Garvey, and Eric Honda. Our clinic nurse Laura Adams kept medical care running throughout the pandemic. Toni Kaulaui, Bernie Ono, and Leslie Boteilho provided heroic service to the community in creating and staffing the North Hawaii Antibody Infusion Clinic.

Queen's administration on both islands assisted me with my move from Punchbowl to North Hawaii, and they also did a fine job of making the hospitals pandemic-proof and facilitating safe discharge for patients. I would like to thank Whitney Lim, Cindy Kamikawa, Yowanda Cortez, Money Atwal, and the late Gary Goldberg for helping to make the relocation of my clinical practice seamless. I'd also like to thank Glenn Rediger and Jill Hoggard Green for taking the quarantine and discharge challenge seriously, making Queen's an early leader in the state on that issue. I owe a particular debt to the Tower 9 nurses at Queen's Punchbowl, and their floor manager Andrea Manaea, for providing me an insight into their challenges delivering care to COVID patients throughout the pandemic.

No success in fighting the pandemic in Hawai'i would have been possible without the efforts of self-organized groups on each island. JoAnn Yukimura, the former mayor of Kaua'i, and Kapono Chong-

Hanssen, the medical director of the Kaua'i Community Health Center, organized one of the largest such efforts on Kaua'i. This group included Chad Taniguchi, Lee Evslin, Phyllis Albert, Steve O'Neal, Mitch Muroff, and Robert Weiner, as well as Professor Michael Schwartz of the University of Washington. Mel Rapozo and Charlie Iona hosted a regular, fact-based broadcast from Kaua'i focused on pandemic issues. An occasional guest on that show was Janet Bereman, the district health officer, whose clear thinking influenced my ideas on the public health response. Dayna Moore's HICOVID group played a similar role on Maui. Chad Meyer, Nicole Ferguson, and Cara Flores were good colleagues and made invaluable contributions on that island. These disparate efforts among the islands merged as the pandemic wore on.

I would like to thank Hiro Toiya, Josh Stanbro, and Georgette Deemer from the City and County of Honolulu, for taking disease control seriously and creating Mayor Caldwell's medical advisory group. On the Big Island, Roy Takemoto performed a similar service for Mayor Kim.

On O'ahu, David Derauf was the person I communicated most frequently with on matters of both policy and science. At the DOH, Libby Char, Eddie Mersereau, and Sarah Kemble were excellent colleagues. At the private micro labs, I'm indebted to Chris Whelen and Owen Chan for numerous and patient discussions of testing technology. Other people with whom I often spoke, and who contributed to my understanding, include Darragh O'Carroll, Gerald S. Murphy, Erick Itoman, Jennifer Frank, Elizabeth Ignacio, James Ireland, Angela Keen, Go Rupal, Scott Miscovich, Kathryn Wong, Josie Howard, Kate Stevens Chang, Dan Escobar, Therese Posas-Mendoza, Daniel Ross, Eric Crawley, Michael Shin, Ajay Bhatt, James Raymond, Jennifer Smith, Liz MacNeill, Graham Taylor, Charles Kick, Aaron Keenan, Mala Arkin, Charles Kohl, George White, Joy Kaaz, Melissa Bolton, Lee Cataluna, Martha Blum, Zubin Damania, Marie Streep, David Watumull, and Patrick Sullivan.

The ideas of numerous thought leaders in academia appear in this book. I owe particular debt to the writing and speaking engagements of Marc Lipsitch, Michael Mina, Trevor Bedford, Shane Crotty, Carl Bergstrom, Paul Offit, Florian Krammer, Dennis Maki, Mark Crislip, Zeynep Tufecki, Sam Harris, Eric Topol, Siddhartha Mukherjee, Mike Ryan, Monica Gandhi, Eran Segal, and Alina Chan.

I want to draw particular attention to Roger Jellinek, an outstanding and patient editor, as well as to his excellent Hawai'i Book and Music Festival, for promoting this book and stimulating a conversation on the state's pandemic response. Likewise, George Engebretson at Watermark Publishing saw the value in this work and made its speedy publication possible.

Most importantly, I would like to thank my family for encouraging me to gather these experiences into a book. Benjamin sat by my side patiently as I read early drafts of chapters. Isaac reminded me not to forget the hydroxychloroquine. My aunt Norma Dapolito was a patient friend over the phone as I worked through various ideas that appear in the book. I want to thank Lance Dworkin, who is my uncle but also my model for what an ethical research scientist in America should stand for. I also want to thank Brad Dworkin, who provided medical care in Westchester through the worst of the epidemic in New York. Michael Schuster and Gayle Goodman gave me masks when they were scarce, and sympathetic ears as the book developed. Andrew Slack encouraged me to get out of my comfort zone as a writer. Aaron Kagan, David Liebesman, and Jordan Hill provided sensible and empathetic advice when I needed it. And I want to thank Layla Schuster, my first editor and best friend, without whose help and support over many years there would be no book, and most likely no infectious diseases doctor to write it.

INTRODUCTION

The ocean is a vast border. Any conversation about pandemics in Hawaiʻi must begin, and perhaps pivot upon, an awareness of this basic geographical fact. For hundreds of years, the Pacific protected Hawaiʻi from epidemic disease. But from their first contact with outsiders, Hawaiians suffered a series of lethal epidemics. Syphilis in 1778. Dysentery in 1804. Pertussis and measles in 1848. Hawaiʻi's population in 1778 was likely four hundred thousand; by 1853, there were only seventy thousand Hawaiians left.

Histories of Hawaiʻi, from the work of O. A. Bushnell to Sumner La Croix, have emphasized the isolation of the Islands and the destruction of the people when that isolation ended. The tragedy that befell the kingdom in the nineteenth century is the backdrop to all contemporary discussion about protecting the health of the Islands. The story of the COVID-19 pandemic occurs downstream from that tragedy. It was the monarchy's response to epidemic disease through the creation of the Queen's Medical Center that made my work, and that of many other doctors, possible.

In 1859, in the wake of a smallpox epidemic, Queen Emma built a hospital on nineteen acres in Honolulu. At that time, the profession of medicine offered only limited insights into microbiology. The project, injured as much by ignorance as by infection, failed to reverse the population decline of the Hawaiian people. But history travels by countercurrents and peculiar eddies. One hundred fifty years later, the Queen's Medical Center survives, now the prized institution of a modern state. Dozens of young doctors from around the world arrive each year to learn a medical science so sophisticated that it would have appeared as magic to the Queen's physicians. The portrait of Emma still hangs in the hall. She watches all, bejeweled, with a glimmer of expectation in her eye. I know the portrait well, because I work in her service, having taken the oath to protect these islands from modern plagues.

The kingdom ravaged and depopulated by epidemics in the nineteenth century became a new Hawai'i that is multicultural, tolerant, and apparently prosperous. The population of Hawai'i is now 1.4 million, with the City and County of Honolulu at just under a million. In genetic terms it's the most diverse population in America, with so much mixing in Hawai'i that there's no clear majority. This fact has profound effects on race relations. Former president Barack Obama grew up on O'ahu in a mixed-race family that placed him within the mainstream of local society. It's notable that he formed his identity as a multiracial American in Hawai'i, while his activism on behalf of Black Americans developed out of his experiences on the Mainland.

The multiculturalism of Hawai'i has a comical side as well. In the winter of 2011, a *New York Times* and Gallup team, perhaps in the depth of seasonal affective despair, built an algorithm to predict happiness. The computer spit back a cryptic solution. The happiest person in America would be a tall man of Chinese ancestry. The man would practice the Jewish faith, own his own business, and reside in Hawai'i. Amused by the terrifying specificity of their oracle, the *Times* team found Alvin Wong, a five-foot, ten-inch Chinese Jew, owner of a healthcare management business in Honolulu, who said that he was indeed extremely satisfied with life.

In 2019, ten million visitors per year were the main driver of Hawai'i's economy, the great majority flying in from Asia and North America. This multibillion-dollar tourism industry directly and indirectly employed close to a third of the residents. If the early monarchs visited the modern city of Honolulu, they would see that it extends for miles beyond its dense urban core, from Koko Head Crater in the east all the way to 'Ewa in the west. On the windward side of O'ahu, they would find the agriculture that defined their era supplanted by the large suburbs of Kailua and Kāne'ohe, and they would encounter a Brigham Young University campus and Mormon temple in Lā'ie. They might be surprised to see people practicing traditional crafts in a reconstructed Polynesian village, not for their own sustenance, but to educate and entertain visitors who had traveled thousands of miles to view the spectacle.

But the wealth and diversity of 2019 concealed an undercurrent of disparity and discontent, and in the years before the pandemic, these problems were becoming increasingly visible. When I returned to the Islands after a fellowship at Brown University, some of my Mainland colleagues imagined that I would spend my days treating exotic infections like leptospirosis and angiostrongylus, the rat lungworm. These are zoonotic pathogens associated with the Islands that are common questions on board exams. But as a Honolulu doctor I encountered an epidemic of infected buttocks wounds. At various times I estimated that as much as a third to half of my patient panel was homeless, a similar percentage had psychiatric or substance-use disorders, and many of these patients were hyper-users of our emergency room. Suffering as much from despair as disease, dozens of these patients practically lived in the hospital, bringing with them a depressing catalogue of skin and soft-tissue pathogens.

In response to this epidemic, which was nothing like the stereotype of medicine in paradise, I reshaped my practice. I began funneling many of my patients through the Queen's Wound Care Center, where two young ER doctors named Michael Shin and Ajay Bhatt were building a practice to meet the city's need. The center provided more comprehensive care for wounds than most patients could get through primary care offices, and by adding infectious diseases, vascular surgery, and plastic surgery components, they provided a multi-specialty service. By 2019, I spent more time in their clinic than in my own office.

The closest thing to a "tropical" pathogen I routinely encountered was *Corynebacterium diphtheriae.* Many people know this as the cause of a toxin-mediated respiratory disease that in previous centuries was fatal for children. Due to a vaccine, that disease has been nearly eradicated. But many people aren't aware that there's a cutaneous ulcer also caused by the bacterium, common in the tropics and associated with poor hygiene and depressed socioeconomic status. I routinely isolated this in the wounds of my homeless patients.

The common infections of Hawaiʻi are diseases of urban blight, and as such say much about the state's social failures.

In 2019, the problems of urban poverty did not seriously threaten the establishment. People who owned homes and businesses profiting from the hospitality industry had little reason to challenge the status quo. Despite the grim evidence of my medical practice, Hawai‘i was a commercial and cultural success, and everywhere I went I saw adverts promoting the aloha spirit. But SARS-CoV-2 would soon disrupt life in ways that went far beyond healthcare, upending assumptions about prosperity and success in Hawai‘i.

The virus exploited the state's inequalities to inflict disproportionate injury on the poorest communities. But it also threatened key institutions—like the hospitals—that everyone relied on. The recession brought on by the pandemic drew attention to the gross disparities in income that had been festering for years. But this economic injury wasn't limited to the poor. The virus shut down entire industries, and it wrecked the long-held consensus, already faltering before the pandemic, that tourism is the best business for Hawai‘i.

I was not the only doctor to struggle against the virus in the shadow of Hawai‘i's history of epidemic disease, or to perceive that the state's geography was a critical asset. I also was not the only person whose work was touched by the growing tension between openness and isolation. I worked closely with a group of friends and colleagues, whom I began to think of as a *hui*. Though we had many connections in healthcare and academia, we had no formal position in the state's governing structures; instead, we used social and traditional media to address and challenge the governing class. At times that class let us in, though it often didn't like what we said. In a few critical moments, however, we persuaded it to alter the course of Hawai‘i's response to the crisis. This is itself an example of the remarkable openness of Hawai‘i, a place in which individuals can breach political barriers and change the direction of a public conversation. Ultimately, Hawai‘i's doctors and nurses, working alongside many others, pushed back the epidemic, while leaving unsolved the problems that made the Islands vulnerable.

These themes became apparent with the passage of time. When I first joined in the state's emergency response, my goal was simply to lift the fog of confusion and help people understand what was coming. I was only dimly aware of the underlying economic and cultural tensions, and I was ignorant of the rules of politics. Had I known, I might have remained silent. But restraint is a virtue I lack, and by time I became aware, our individual desires were irrelevant. We were in the grip of history. ☙

Chapter One

EMERGENCE

JANUARY 31, 2020

0

HAWAIʻI

6	9,826
UNITED STATES	WORLD

COVID-19 cases (data sources: World Health Organization and Hawaii Department of Health)

The first time I heard Dennis Maki speak was a dreary afternoon in August 2012, not long after I finished my infectious diseases fellowship. I was plowing through dozens of lectures to prepare for my board exams. Even after years of clinical training, no physician sees every disease. But the boards expect you to know everything, so you spend many hours brushing up on arcane infections that you may encounter once or twice in the course of a career.

Maki's lecture caught my interest, and one slide in particular etched itself in my brain. He described his own decision to become an infectious diseases doctor—and the concern this caused in his mentors. At the time, infections were on their way out. Pasteurization, sterile surgical technique, vaccination, and antibiotics had, by the middle of the twentieth century, consigned infections to the history books. Or so it seemed. Maki's advisors thought a talented young man was ill-advised to waste his time studying historical curiosities when there were exciting advances in cardiology to pursue.

Maki broke out his best slide. It's a simple slide. It lists new infections discovered during the course of the past four decades, and shows the year of emergence. Some of the infections are obscure to most readers. Nipah virus? Unless you work with date palm sap, you probably aren't familiar with that one. But others, like HIV, exploded through human populations and changed the course of history. More alarmingly, the rate of emergence of new infections accelerated as the twentieth century waned. By 2010, the world averaged a new or re-emergent pathogen every year. Far from studying an obscure topic, Maki found himself at the center of the fastest-growing field in medicine.

How did this happen? How did infectious diseases go from being nearly a dead subspecialty to the most important on the planet? And why did so many smart people fail to predict this?

Emergence is the discovery of new infections causing epidemic disease, or an increase in incidence or geographic range of a previously discovered infection. The key to understanding emergence is to look skeptically at human behavior. Nature is a great library of species, too immense for humans to catalog, let alone memorize. When you venture into nature, you pick a book off a shelf and begin leafing through the pages. You encounter thousands of species each day; the vast majority of them are microscopic, and many of them are a part of your own body. Most of these are harmless to you. Many species (for example, bacteria that aid in digestion) are essential for your survival. But each species evolves to fill a niche, and when you disturb that niche, you create an opportunity for a novel interaction between yourself and the microbe.

Some try to differentiate between "good" and "bad" microbes, the good label generally denoting a symbiotic relationship between human and microbe. But this doesn't quite capture the dynamic. Even a "good" bacteria can cause infection if its normal ecology is disturbed. For example, *Escherichia coli* in the large intestine aids in the synthesis of vitamin K. However, in diseases where there's a disturbance of the luminal barrier of the gut (e.g., diverticulitis), *E. coli* can enter the bloodstream and cause overwhelming sepsis. To add an additional wrinkle, patients exposed to antibiotics will develop multi-drug resistant variants of *E. coli*. Most of the time, the hardier *E. coli* will behave just like the old, sensitive ones. They will inhabit the gut, contribute to the person's biochemistry, and reproduce. But given an opportunity to invade, they will, and they carry with them the multidrug resistant phenotype that physicians bestowed on them by exposure to the antibiotic. These infections carry a higher risk of death.

Emergence, therefore, is the result of microbial opportunity, and opportunity happens most often when human behavior shifts. And this is why emergence as a concept doesn't just apply to novel microbes. Well-known microbes can re-emerge due to changes in society. When the Soviet Union collapsed in 1990, the country experienced the largest outbreak of diphtheria to impact any industrialized country in decades. The relevant factors in that epidemic were urban crowding, population movement, and a decrease in timely vaccine coverage for children. A disease long-thought dead roared back as the microbe filled a new niche created by poverty and social upheaval.

When I teach medical students and residents about emergence, I encourage them to think about their daily economy. How much of their day is spent in human-created spaces that have resulted from some perturbation of the environment? What resources are they consuming, and what's required from nature to generate these resources?

I live in a house built on land that was once a forest. My breakfast eggs come from a farm that is mass producing chickens. I try to buy local eggs and from farms that treat their animals well. But I am trusting labels. Often enough I eat a factory egg produced by a chicken that has been crowded into a pen like a prisoner in a concentration camp. My poor bird is exposed to thousands of other birds. The clothes I wear may be synthetic, and some of the compounds used in shipping them have antimicrobial properties that interact with my own flora. When I go to the hospital to work, I am entering the most artificial environment created by humans. This is a place where every surface material is synthetic, to aid in cleaning. During the course of a day, I put plastic catheters into my patients' veins, order surgical procedures, and prescribe them drugs that alter their immunity. The hospital contains hundreds of people whose lives are being prolonged by intense human intervention. They share rooms, share nurses, and breathe the same air. Is it any surprise that the most aggressive pathogens on the planet evolved to fill this niche?

So maybe the Luddites are right. Maybe modern society contains within it the kernel of its own demise, and the emergence of infectious diseases is merely one form of the reaper.

To better visualize these interactions, I share with the students a graphic of my own making.

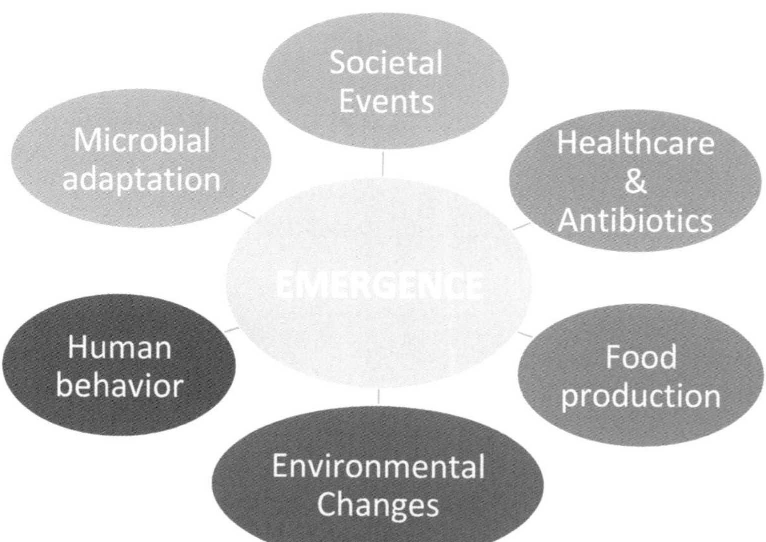

Figure 1.1 Factors leading to the emergence of infectious diseases

It's the combination of two or more of these variables that most often accounts for emergence of a new infection, or re-emergence of an old one. And the key to understanding the acceleration of discovery of new pathogens is in the observation that our society, as it becomes more technically sophisticated, has exponentially increased its impact on these variables.

Dengue fever spread throughout the world as a result of its host mosquito hitching a ride on Allied shipping during World War II, with large outbreaks occurring in urbanizing areas during the postwar years. To take a more mundane example, coagulase-negative staphylococcus species are ubiquitous in the environment, often living on human skin. They weren't considered pathogens until about fifty years ago. They became pathogens when doctors began putting prosthetic material in people as part of joint replacement surgery, heart valve replacement surgery, and central venous catheter procedures. The HIV epidemic originated in Africa, likely as a result of people harvesting bush meat. That's an intrusion into the environment. But it spread as a result of global trade and changes in sexual mores.

The lessons of emergence are clear. New opportunities for microbial adaptation, most often created by human behavior, lead to new or re-emergent infectious diseases. Emergence happens naturally, and not just in humans. But the growth in human population and the increased impact on the environment through industry and technology have led to an acceleration in emergence. And this leads to the second major lesson I can glean from this history, which is that the human response, itself a set of behaviors, is the key to containing epidemics.

I became aware of the novel coronavirus around New Year's 2020, at the same time as millions of other people, when reports surfaced of a new respiratory illness sickening patients in Wuhan, China. I clicked through the news items with some interest. Shortly afterwards, an electron micrograph picture was published showing the characteristic "crown" of a coronavirus. I remember showing the picture to my sons and making an offhand remark, something like "Would you like to see a picture of the world's newest infectious disease?" There was limited enthusiasm. My kids are used to this kind of provocation from their dad. But there was some curiosity about this picture, the virus made visible to human eyes, its ominous spikes emerging like a medieval battlement.

I was in medical school during the original SARS outbreak, and I gave a lecture at Queen's on emergence of infections during the MERS epidemic. A novel coronavirus was a surprise to no one. But the experiences with SARS and MERS lulled the medical profession to complacency. Both of those epidemics caused severe symptoms in patients who were infected. Neither was highly contagious. Because the cases were more easily identified, the resulting epidemics were more easily contained. There had been little global research on coronavirus treatments, and there was no vaccine candidate "on the shelf" that could be rapidly mobilized. Too much pandemic preparedness assumed that influenza would be the pathogen, and influenza proved an imperfect analogy.

The debate over how the coronavirus emerged may remain unsettled for years, perhaps forever given the secrecy of the Chinese state. Initially, the government made attempts to downplay the significance of the outbreak. They threatened whistleblowers, including the Chinese ophthalmologist Li Wenliang, who died of the disease. The Chinese rapidly sequenced the genome but failed to share their data in a timely way. In January, the sequence became public information. Experts in virology analyzed the genome and placed it on a phylogenetic map, locating it as a cousin of the original SARS virus. The science of genotyping has progressed enormously in recent years, and it's not difficult to compare new genomes to existing ones known from nature or lab work. The genome's closest relative is a species found in bats in a rural province of China. Early cases in the Wuhan seafood market suggested emergence as a result of some interaction between bats and humans, possibly through an intermediate animal. This fit nicely with the story of the original SARS, which also emerged from bats and used palm civets as the intermediate host.

This explanation was incomplete, though, and in truth the rush by scientists to label the virus of zoonotic origin was premature. The Wuhan seafood market was an early superspreader event (i.e., a place where one case became many), and this is why it drew attention, but the disease likely circulated for weeks previously. It's now clear that there were early cases with no ties to the outbreak in that venue. This places the point of emergence earlier, most likely in October–November 2019.

Interestingly, no intermediate animal host was found, nor were animal samples at the seafood market positive for virus, facts that make markets and agriculture a less likely explanation for emergence. But more concerning than the lack of a clear environmental origin for the virus is the secrecy of the Chinese government, which shut down research into the origin of the virus. That dovetails with reports in American newspapers that the Wuhan Institute of Virology not only worked with coronaviruses but had been identified as a source of biohazard risk in a State Department cable in 2018. Could the virus have escaped from the lab through human error?

There are precedents for this. Dystopian Hollywood scripts aside, it turns out that humans are quite inept at containing dangerous pathogens in scientific facilities. A Russian lab strain of influenza caused an influenza epidemic in 1977, mostly forgotten because the disease was mild. Biosafety failures in the United Kingdom released foot and mouth disease in 2007. Investigations have revealed hundreds of reports of lab handling errors in biosafety level 3 and 4 labs, which contain the most transmissible and deadly pathogens. Given the known risks and documented lab failures, and in particular the behavior of the Chinese government, a lab escape theory for SARS-CoV-2 can't be excluded.

Alina Chan, a postdoc at the Broad Institute of MIT and Harvard, has raised the most prominent concerns about lab escape at the Wuhan Institute of Virology. The issue revolves around a strain of coronavirus known as RaTG13, which is the closest known matching virus to SARS-CoV-2. The genome for RaTG13 was published after the pandemic began. But Chan points out that RaTG13 is the same virus as a previously identified coronavirus known as BtCoV/4991. This is important, because BtCoV/4991 was sequenced in 2018, two years before the pandemic. And who were the sequencers? The Wuhan Institute of Virology. The BtCoV/4991 virus had been isolated from a mine shaft in Yunnan, China, in 2013, not long after miners became ill with a viral respiratory illness.

It was sleuths like Chan, working through the data and collaborating online, who revealed that this virus was present in the Wuhan lab, and that Chinese scientists sequenced it before the pandemic. The scientists in

Wuhan insist there's nothing amiss here, and that they never cultured the virus (a process that would increase the chances of a mishap). But without access to their lab, the rest of the world is taking their word for it. No one outside the Chinese government, and perhaps a few scientists working on their coronavirus program, knows how many other viruses they sampled, sequenced, cultured, or altered.

These activities, including the creation of "chimeric" viruses (in which parts of one virus are combined with parts of another to assess infectiousness), occurred at the Wuhan Institute of Virology. Much confusion has resulted from the argument over whether this research—which the institute carried out in the open and in collaboration with American co-investigators—meets the definition of "gain of function." That term has become synonymous in the public imagination with unsafe lab experiments on pathogens. Arguably, the Wuhan work did not, as the purpose was to assess the potential for a given animal virus (as opposed to a known human pathogen) to spill over into the human population. The case for conducting these experiments, which arose in the wake of the SARS-CoV-1 epidemic, was presented as defensive in nature (i.e., to better understand the science of spillover and define the risk to public health). But given the potential for such experiments to generate new variants that may spread to humans, it's a distinction that could be moot. And without an audit of the lab, we can't know the extent of such research, whether mishaps occurred, or whether the Chinese government authorized more dangerous experiments that never saw the light of peer review.

Ironically, it was the American government that muddied the culpability of Chinese labs in beginning the pandemic. Not only did anti-Chinese sentiment infiltrate the thinking and rhetoric of senior government officials, including the president, but political operatives working parallel to the White House vastly overstated the case for lab origins by publicizing a discredited hypothesis alleging that SARS-CoV-2 was a bioweapon. Aside from the fact that there's no credible evidence to support this assertion, an intentional release had the Chinese deploying the weapon first in their own city, a mere few hundred yards from their principal virology facility. That's an act so stupid and self-incriminating that it's hard to take seriously.

Unlike the hypothesis of accidental release, the bioweapons

explanation had far more to do with politics than science. It rested on the claims made by Li-Meng Yan, a whistleblower from Hong Kong seeking political asylum in the United States. Yan was dependent on Guo Wengui, a businessman in exile from China, as well as Steve Bannon, the former Trump advisor. Bannon was later indicted for conspiracy to commit wire fraud, based on fundraising for Trump's border wall that prosecutors alleged was diverted for his own use. The arrest occurred on Wengui's $35 million yacht. Prior to leaving office, Trump pardoned Bannon. But despite the shady patronage of her claims, and the fact that most virologists disputed her hypothesis on technical grounds, Yan's arguments were widely circulated in right wing media. By attacking the Chinese government in such a clumsy way, the American right empowered them to dismiss any lab-leak investigation as an expression of anti-Chinese chauvinism.

In the struggle between the two powers, this failure of American propaganda ended with a World Health Organization (WHO) investigation of SARS-CoV-2 emergence in January and February of 2021. Reflecting the decline of American prestige within international institutions, and the nation's exit from the WHO in 2020, the investigation occurred in the friendliest context possible for the Chinese. The timing, a full year after the pandemic began, increased the odds that nothing controversial would be uncovered. A rigorous and independent investigation at the time of the outbreak would have allowed earlier and more accurate contact tracing, environmental sampling, analysis of blood bank samples, and most importantly, an audit of the laboratory.

Instead, origins-related data shared with the WHO team was curated by the Chinese government, which had months to prepare for the visit. There was no investigation of the Wuhan lab. One member of the WHO team, Peter Daszak, was so compromised by prior financial relationships with his counterparts in Wuhan that he had already announced, a mere weeks after the pandemic began, that lab origin theories should be dismissed. The team consisted only of members acceptable to the Chinese government. They lacked the mandate to investigate lab origins, yet unwisely agreed to a press conference with the Chinese, during which they dismissed the idea. That was a win for the host government. The team also endorsed the Chinese talking point that SARS-CoV-2 may have originated in frozen food imports from China's Southeast Asian neighbors, encouraging the next investigation to occur far from Wuhan.

Despite this unsteady attempt at reassurance, the team leader acknowledged, after leaving China, that they had no real basis for discounting lab origins. Members of the team admitted they were under intense political pressure during their visit, and they found no concrete evidence of an environmental origin for the virus.

The controversy over the Wuhan lab is real, but that doesn't mean that lab escape is the origin of SARS-CoV-2. The RaTG13 genome is 96 percent similar to SARS-CoV-2, but 4 percent difference is a lot. The 4 percent gap is most suggestive of the two viruses sharing a common ancestor decades ago. Emergence from a population of bats remains possible, and the absence of a known natural exposure is not evidence that one never occurred. If it emerged in nature, it's likely that the first cases went unrecognized, and the wider outbreak in Wuhan that occurred some weeks later became the incorrect origin point in early news reports. It's also possible that emergence has an agricultural origin, with an intermediate species not yet identified, although how the virus appeared hundreds or thousands of miles distant in Wuhan without leaving a trail through the food production industry remains unclear.

Some of my colleagues wish to downplay the controversy over the origins of SARS-CoV-2. In terms of medical management, it doesn't matter whether the pandemic arose from natural exposure, agriculture, or lab escape. But I disagree with this passivity. Just as human behavior led to emergence, the early response of humans amplified the epidemic. The mildest judgment that can be made about the Chinese government is that their attempted cover-up made the pandemic far more likely. There's a heavy toll of suffering that can be felt as a consequence of their disregard for their own people and their neighbors.

Without a clear picture of emergence, governments can't mitigate the risk of a future pandemic, which is why China's unwillingness to work towards a better understanding of how SARS-CoV-2 emerged is not just suspicious, it's dangerous. The American attempt to leverage that controversy politically, which was crude and demagogic, should not distract anyone from the underlying issue. As Alina Chan has argued, without a credible investigation of the lab, governments around the world will be empowered to continue potentially dangerous research, secure in the knowledge that as long as they don't publish their samples, they can obstruct any subsequent inquiry. The result is a world in which engineered viruses aren't merely a theoretical possibility, but an ongoing part of our political and military landscape. ☙

Chapter Two

KOREA, ITALY, AND IRAN

FEBRUARY 29, 2020

0	
HAWAIʻI	
62	85,403
UNITED STATES	WORLD

COVID-19 cases (data sources: World Health Organization and Hawaii Department of Health)

In January, I became worried. My wife was in India, traveling with friends from New York. She had to travel back to Honolulu through connections in New Delhi and Tokyo. The news from China that month progressed from curious to alarming. The outbreak in Wuhan was out of control, and I was particularly concerned to see a smattering of cases in neighboring countries such as Vietnam, Singapore, and Japan. I still didn't have clear information about the extent of the problem inside China, about contagiousness, or about the mortality rate. But the increasingly drastic lockdown in Wuhan spoke for itself.

I began at this time a daily ritual that I credit with keeping my mind clear during what became a blizzard of conflicting and often erroneous information. Each day, I visited the WHO website and recorded the number of cases outside China. I thought that due to the chaos in Wuhan—and related attempts by the government to control information—any data from within China would be intrinsically unreliable. But if the case counts began to rise in neighboring countries, that would be alarming. In particular, I defined a logarithmic rise in non-China cases occurring over a period of a week or two (i.e., the expected interval between cases) to be an unambiguous red flag.

At this early point, I assumed that the spread would occur within China's contiguous neighbors, and I thought that India was at high risk for a respiratory virus, given its population density. This was half right, but I was about six months early, and I still didn't understand how variables like age and seasonality would impact the progression of the disease. I spent a lot of time worrying about my wife and her airport connections, but she arrived home safely at the end of January.

In the meantime, my graph showed a steady trickle of cases outside China. Singapore had an especially reliable public health system and faithfully reported its cases daily. Their data showed a stubborn tendency of cases to crop up in clusters after a few days of quiet. The authorities in Singapore were well prepared and responded aggressively, but they couldn't eradicate transmission altogether. Likewise, the Japanese reported a small but steady increase in cases throughout the month. This indicated that containment within Wuhan was failing, and that neighboring countries with excellent health sectors were struggling to eradicate the virus.

I had numerous conversations with colleagues at this time, including Masayuki Nogi, an excellent internist at Queen's with academic connections in Japan. We both felt that travel restrictions were appropriate, and that the likelihood we would see containment in the US as robust as that in Japan or Singapore was low. Japan, with its numerous air links to both China and the US, and its slowly rising case count, was an early focus of our attention.

But the virus had different plans, and it was with some surprise in mid-February that I noted large new clusters forming in Korea, Italy, and Iran. The Korean epidemic was quickly linked to a religious group that had travel contacts to China. But the Italian and Iranian outbreaks were more mysterious. This was the first of many surprises that the new virus delivered.

I was soon to become used to shocking and seemingly random eruptions of cases. I didn't yet understand the mechanics of virus transmission. I assumed that transmission would follow from a source country to its neighbors. I soon learned that much transmission was asymptomatic, and that most transmission chains dead-end, but a few propagate. There is an element of chance in this, with increased air connections leading to higher odds of sustained transmission in a given place. The virologist Trevor Bedford has described this as analogous to embers being blown off a bonfire. The exact place a spark lands is random, though it is influenced by the winds. And most embers don't cause secondary fires; they simply die out. But a few will, and the longer you allow the bonfire to burn uninterrupted, the more secondary blazes you will find downwind.

The three new countries fell into crisis, with clusters of a few dozen patients rapidly becoming hundreds and then thousands of cases. This dwarfed in scale anything previously seen, and Japan quickly lost its ignoble ranking as the second-most-infected country on my daily graph. The authorities in Wuhan had, by February, begun to get the upper hand on their epidemic. But the Chinese had locked down hundreds of millions of people, cutting off road and rail links to Hubei province and mobilizing an army of healthcare providers and relief workers. The level of government suppression remained high, and the sheer scale of their effort was unlike anything contemplated in democratic countries.

The Korean outbreak destroyed any remaining illusions I may have held about containing the disease to China. Korea experienced a trickle of cases in late January and early February, similar to other countries near China. But on February 20, they reported seventy new cases. This dramatic increase was due to one of the first well-documented superspreader events, a congregant who attended church in the town of Daegu after becoming symptomatic. The Daegu cluster occurred among the Shincheonji Church of Jesus, a group known for large gatherings and lack of physical spacing. By the end of February, Korea had over two thousand confirmed cases.

This menace, growing like a metastasis outside of China, prompted a heavy government response, with movement restrictions imposed on Daegu and many daily activities around the country canceled. But what differentiated the Korean response was its elegant and timely use of technology to control the outbreak. With the church serving as the epicenter of infection, contact tracing was successful in identifying many of the downstream exposures. The Koreans deployed molecular testing to differentiate infected people from uninfected. These companies were local, and they continued to provide the government with a high level of service even when testing resources became strained in other countries. The Korean disease control effort made use of cellular phone and credit card data to track the movement of confirmed cases. They quickly built a system of government-supported shelters to isolate and support patients so that they wouldn't infect their family members. By April, Korea had flattened its epidemic curve, and I began looking to them as a model of disease containment.

Around this time, in early spring, I watched a video online that illustrated the success of the Korean containment system. A young man named Kim Jaehan returned to Korea after travel abroad. A hotline took his travel history. The operator instructed him to get a test. He related that he didn't have his own car to drive to the testing center. No problem: an ambulance with a fiberglass divide between the driver and rear seats arrived to take him. At the testing center, the tech swabbed the back of his nose and his throat. He then produced a sputum sample. The center sent all three samples for a molecular test, and the ambulance took him home. During the next twenty-four hours, he was provided food at his door. At one point he received a call from the quarantine operator, who scolded him because his phone was off. He explained he wasn't out walking; it just turned off. She told him to leave it on. If she couldn't see that he was in the apartment, she would have to call the police to check on him. Later, his test returned negative, but he was told to continue a fourteen-day home quarantine.

What's notable about the Korean response is the integration of the different components of disease control. There was a hotline to collect information and coordinate services. That, in turn, was tied to the transport service, a test center, a mobile app for tracking, and quarantine services. There were five moving parts here, but it's their synergy that made the system work.

Other countries would soon devise disease-control systems that were highly successful and relied on components of the Korean model. Over the subsequent few months, Taiwan, Hong Kong, Vietnam, and New Zealand all experienced sustained success in keeping cases down. No two systems were precisely the same, and strategies varied by geography and local culture. But certain elements were constant in all successful SARS-CoV-2 control models. Border control, particularly for islands, was critical. The Koreans made liberal use of testing, and the Vietnamese were more resource-limited, but both tied testing to contact tracing and isolation of cases. In most successful countries, a centralized isolation and quarantine, with the government assigning rooms and ensuring enforcement, was a key plank. The most critical variable was social cohesion. Governments that were honest created buy-in from the public, who then self-policed and ensured high rates of adherence to the public health strategy.

Italy and Iran were not as well prepared. The Italian epidemic hit in the north, with Bergamo at its epicenter. Many residents were elderly, and multigenerational families were common. Physicians there followed a WHO protocol that restricted testing to patients with a confirmed China travel history, a fidelity that proved disastrous, as the virus was already circulating. The government delayed its response, based in part on industry pressure, and the inevitable lockdown came too late. As *The Guardian* reported:

> The Italian government had declared a nationwide health emergency on 31 January but Stefano Scaglia, the president of Confindustria Bergamo, which represents 1,200 businesses employing 80,000 people, offered reassurance. On 29 February, the organization published a message in English aimed at the region's international export partners, accompanied by the hashtag

> "#Bergamoisrunning." Drawing on the Italian government's advice it said "the risk of infection is low" and warned against "a distorted perception" created by the media. Confindustria could guarantee that "the government and responsible agencies have taken immediate protective measures to prevent further cases."

This was the opposite of Korean candor. And it's a dark irony that a strong work ethic proved to be the undoing of the Italians. The easier-going southern provinces fared well. But in the north, within weeks Italy would be using its army to transport corpses. Large daily case numbers continued well into April. The hospitals became overwhelmed, and the mortality rate amongst confirmed cases reached 10 percent. As in Wuhan, much of the excess mortality occurred because ICU services were saturated and staff fell ill.

Iran fared no better. With limited ICU and public health resources, satellite images of mass graves began appearing in the American papers. In early March, a physician friend from the Kurdish region sent me a video of an Iranian hospital morgue filled with bodies. Italy eventually contained its outbreak with a lockdown, but cases and fatalities in Iran remained high for months, and they seeded additional large outbreaks in Iraq and the Gulf states.

The Iranian outbreak had sequelae that were of personal interest. I had long-standing ties with physician colleagues in the Kurdish region. The Kurds are a stateless people, deprived of independence by the politicking of the Allies following World War I. They are spread over a mountainous border area that divides the modern states of Turkey, Syria, Iraq, and Iran. The Kurdish region in northern Iraq is autonomous. It's also a key American ally, and I have friends there dating back to medical visits organized during my student days.

The Kurdish struggle against the virus illustrates the problems with containment of a respiratory pathogen. Kurdish physicians in Duhok published a series of early cases in March and April. The series showed travel ties with European countries, but with subsequent transmission to close contacts in the region. The Kurds responded aggressively, imposing a brief curfew in their capital Erbil, followed by a general lockdown. Due to this response, they largely eliminated the early transmission chains. For several weeks in March and April, they enjoyed great success, despite the unfolding catastrophe across the border in Iran. Friends sent me a video of a young man receiving a short-cropped haircut, popular in the region, with Kurdish pop music playing in the background. The barber attached his razor to a long stick and conducted the operation from a distance of six feet.

Perennial underdogs, Kurds relished these low-tech solutions. But months later, in June, the comedy ended. The virus came roaring back in the form of a large outbreak in Sulaimania. This was a curious occurrence, as cases in the other Kurdish provinces, as well as the rest of Iraq, lagged behind. Sulaimania is the city I worked in, and it's where my friends live. A college town, it's known in Iraq for its history of poets and its liberal politics. But it's also known for its economic dependence on cross-border trade with Iran, some of which coasts beneath the bounds of legality. Trade and smuggling aside, many Kurds on the Iraqi side of the border travel to Iran for school or for healthcare. These arrangements could not be permanently halted, and it's likely the virus entered the region through this travel or alongside some untaxed contraband.

Within a few weeks, Sulaimania had thousands of cases, and the local press was comparing the healthcare situation to that which occurred earlier in Italy. It was a vivid demonstration of the difficulties in keeping a respiratory pathogen at bay. The Kurds have a saying, "our only friends are the mountains." But high terrain was no obstacle to SARS-CoV-2. The virus crossed mountains, just as it had penetrated airports and seaports elsewhere, finding its way across a porous border where trade imperatives took precedence over disease control.

As February progressed, there was confusion in the United States. President Trump downplayed the threat, uttering his infamous "it miraculously goes away" line on February 10 at a campaign event in New Hampshire. He doubled down on February 24, tweeting, "The Coronavirus is very much under control in the USA." On March 11, in an Oval Office address, he reiterated, "The risk is very, very low." A few days later, on March 19, in an interview with Bob Woodward for his book *Rage*, he admitted, "I wanted to always play it down. I still like playing it

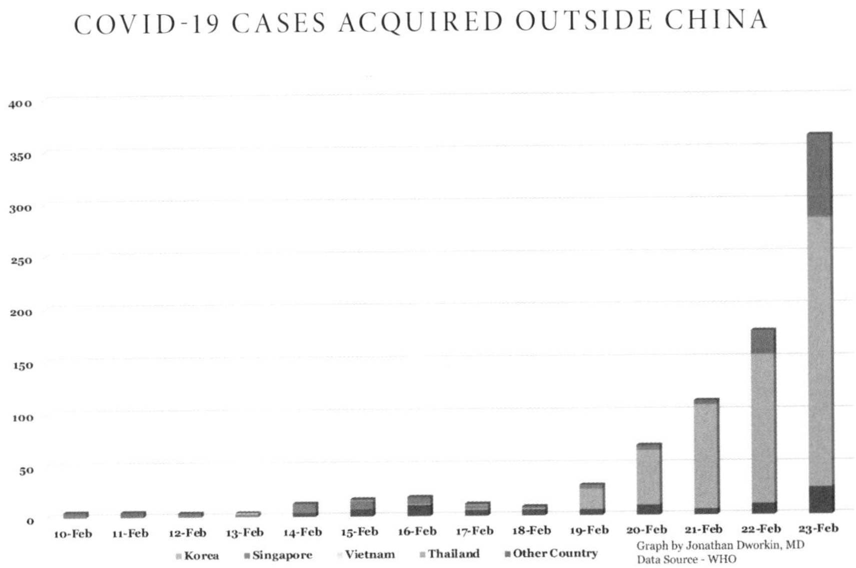

Figure 2.1 An early graph by author showing cases outside China

down, because I don't want to create a panic." Trump's irresponsibility echoed misstatements from the Centers for Disease Control (CDC). On January 31, the CDC director, Robert Redfield, said, "I want to emphasize that the risk to the American public is currently low."

Contrast this with Jacinda Ardern, the prime minister of New Zealand. On February 2, she announced that any foreign traveler from or passing through China would be denied entry to New Zealand. This action was coordinated with the Australian prime minister, and it was consistent with American travel restrictions. But with the disease spreading, on March 14, she announced much tougher border controls, including a mandatory fourteen-day quarantine for everyone coming into New Zealand. She concluded:

> [W]e have two choices as a nation. One is to let COVID-19 roll on, and brace. The second is to go hard on measures to keep it out, and stamp it out.... I make no apology for choosing the second path. New Zealanders' public health comes first. If we have that, we can recover from the impacts on the

economy, the impacts on tourism, and the impacts on our airline.

This gives the lie to the common claim that success against the virus was a product of the more hierarchical Asian culture, and that no such coordinated effort could be expected in Western countries. The implication, convenient for people who had already embraced fatalism in the struggle against the virus, is that American virtues like individualism made a coherent and effective response impossible. But New Zealand and Australia both benefited from an aggressive government response despite a strong libertarian streak in their cultures, especially in Australia. Scandinavian countries, with the exception of Sweden, also did well. Germany and Canada performed an order of magnitude better than the United States in disease control. The difference was the willingness of powerful people in those countries to speak plainly about the threat and to request help from their people.

Dishonest messaging was only one of America's issues. Technical and organizational setbacks were soon to cripple the CDC's early containment efforts. Unlike the Koreans, the United States had no private labs approved to test patients. That required overcoming a regulatory obstacle at the Food and Drug Administration (FDA). Under ordinary circumstances, the CDC develops a test and makes it available through state departments of health, who in turn control access to testing. As private labs build capacity, they apply for FDA approval, at which point test kits become more widely available to the public. However, events happened so fast in February that it soon became obvious there was no time for this ponderous process. Even worse, the CDC kit failed, leaving the health departments blind. As the CDC struggled to resolve its technical problems, the FDA maintained its nonsensical restrictions on the private labs. The end result was that the United States had no idea whether transmission had begun in this country. But that didn't stop federal officials from falsely reassuring everyone.

Another early failure occurred with the evacuation of US citizens from Wuhan and from virus-afflicted cruise ships. Territorial battles between federal agencies precluded coordinated effort to repatriate Americans. In one well-described case, hundreds of passengers from the *Costa Luminosa* cruise ship boarded commercial flights in Atlanta, despite dozens of confirmed cases on that ship. The CDC described their policy as follows:

> For well travelers, it is part of CDC's protocol to recommend that they continue expeditiously on flights home following disembarkation from cruise ships and chartered flights back to the US.... We gave passengers information at the airport about how to monitor their health, and advised them to immediately quarantine for 14 days after they arrive home.

If the CDC believed these people needed to quarantine, then it made no sense to put them on commercial flights. The result was that many passengers became sick in the middle of their flights, and the federal government airmailed the virus around the country. Even now, the scale and consequences of this error aren't fully known, because many passengers were no longer subject to federal scrutiny after returning home. But there's reason to believe this was no small mistake. A CDC report from late March documented hundreds of cases on dozens of cruise ships, accounting for almost 20 percent of known cases during the first month of the US epidemic.

The cruise ship mess reflected a deeper unwillingness on the part of the CDC to lead. As later reporting would show, other federal agencies intended to defer to the CDC on infection control policies. But the CDC insisted that each federal agency must be responsible for its handling of repatriated Americans. This led to infection control failures at the March Air Reserve Base in California, where the federal government housed evacuees from Wuhan. The country needed a centralized structure in which CDC brains informed military brawn to produce an efficient evacuation and re-entry system. Instead, interagency turf struggles hobbled the American response and became a conduit by which the virus entered the country.

Denial wasn't merely an activity for politicians and public health officers. Prominent physicians, including Zubin Damania, who has a comedic and influential presence on social media, were more concerned by public panic than government ineptitude. But I didn't see people panicking. It was our failure to prepare for the disease that was the imminent threat, and the shortcomings of our prostrate response were increasingly evident. This was an instructive example of the psychology of risk. In most cases, people warning of imminent catastrophe are crazy. But February 2020 was an inversion of the usual dynamic. Those of us drawing attention to the noose tightening around our necks were, in that brief and confusing interlude, the only sober ones.

As I learned during subsequent reading, there's a long history of dishonest communication around epidemics in America. During the 1918 influenza pandemic, President Wilson refused to talk about the disease. He viewed it as a distraction from the war effort against Germany. Newspapers around the country instead repeated fake reassurances from local officials. "Don't panic" was the most common advice. When people realized the scale of the threat, panic gripped entire cities, and officials no longer enjoyed any public confidence.

The two stupidest words uttered in February and March of 2020 were "don't panic." The four stupidest words were "the risk is low." Both phrases were repeated endlessly, with the leaden stubbornness of groupthink. This sanguine propaganda was in perfect—and for the most part subconscious—symmetry with the disastrous pandemic playbook of 1918. The phrases were a near-certain marker of denial. It would have been far better for officials at every level to paint a grim picture for the public, so that people understood they were expected to make some sacrifices for the common good. This was, after all, the successful approach taken by the authorities in Korea and New Zealand. But such an effort in America would have required foresight and courage, which proved to be in even shorter supply than masks and tests.

During the events in Korea, Italy, and Iran, it became clear to me that the coronavirus from Wuhan would spread around the world. On leap day, in a post shared on Facebook, I first used the word "pandemic," though I had been contemplating the word for some time. I wrote at length about why the threat to the United States was real:

> If you look at the measures being taken in countries heavily impacted by the new virus in order to control it, what you see is a level of disruption that few people alive are accustomed to. Prolonged closures of public spaces. Quarantines of entire towns. A massive decrease in air travel and public transit. What this amounts to is a major disruption in cultural and economic activity. And those measures seem to be slowing, but not stopping, spread of the virus.

I had contact with many people in the medical community in Hawai'i dating back years to my internal medicine training and subsequent private practice work. The Facebook post was useful because it expressed out loud what a lot of people were beginning to worry in private. As such, it was a well-timed conversation starter. The post received far more attention than anything I had written previously. Many people expressed relief, both in public and private, to receive honest information. Not long afterwards, James Ireland, a nephrologist I worked with during my training, and who worked with the airport on emergency medical response, invited me to join the lieutenant governor's weekly phone calls.

This was the beginning of my association with Hawai'i's containment effort, and it was my introduction to people in the state's government and business circles. It proved an awkward fit. I soon learned the wisdom of Upton Sinclair's famous remark that "it is difficult to get a man to understand something, when his salary depends on him not understanding it." The same could be said for power. But on the leap day, the inanity of local politics was far from my mind. I wanted only to ring the warning bell. ☙

Chapter Three

AN EERIE QUIET

MARCH 31, 2020

283	
HAWAIʻI	
140,640	750,890
UNITED STATES	WORLD

COVID-19 cases (data sources: World Health Organization and Hawaii Department of Health)

February and early March passed in Hawaiʻi with little change, at least on the surface. With the exception of Chinese tourists, now absent, visitors flooded in from around the world and enjoyed beaches, bars, and national parks. The tourism engine was insatiable, and as had become common in pre-pandemic months, the state hosted close to a million travelers. But by now it was apparent that the state's economic lifeline was a threat to its existence. The virus must reach Hawaiʻi through transpacific travel, as there was no other way for it to get in. Given the visitor numbers from East Asia, I thought an introduction from Japan, Singapore, or Korea was most likely. Little did I know that the virus was already spreading widely on the US Mainland.

One of the most difficult aspects of dealing with the new virus was the inversion in normal thinking required to counter it. For decades, the foundation of wealth in Hawai'i was an openness to the outside world. The entire economic and social structure was built on this idea of welcoming people from all over the globe. Residents now had to grapple with the notion that hosting visitors would introduce a deadly infection, but locking them out would mean placing in deep freeze a half-century of economic progress.

This had implications beyond the economy. Casual observers often assume aloha is insincere, or a marketing ploy, and it's true that some local companies have used it for branding in ways that dilute its meaning. But for people raised in the Islands, aloha is a serious idea. It's a concept that connotes not just welcoming but generosity, and handled respectfully, aloha reflects one's own internal state of graciousness.

It shouldn't surprise anyone that Hawai'i struggled with these problems, largely ignoring them during February and early March. Business continued as usual, despite the worrying rise in my daily graphs of cases outside China.

In truth, the problems were deeper than a mere resistance to the changing reality. The pattern of denial that unfolded nationally cast its mirror image at the state level in Hawai'i's political scene. The first mention of the virus in an official Hawaii Department of Health (DOH) communication came on January 29. Stating that "the risk to the general public is low," the DOH nonetheless reassured the public that they investigated all possible cases quickly. The first statement was untrue, and the second proved beyond their ability.

A later DOH communication on February 14 described the first known case in Hawai'i, a Japanese national who visited Maui from January 28 to February 3, as well as O'ahu from February 3 to 7. He became symptomatic while on O'ahu. "The individual had no symptoms on Maui and was not contagious," said Dr. Sarah Park, the state epidemiologist. The press release ended with a message for everyone to get their flu shot. Maui officials further tried to calm their residents. "This is not the time to panic," said Lee Weiss, the medical director at Maui Memorial. "Here at Maui Memorial Medical Center, we have comprehensive plans in place and are being very vigilant in our screening and care of patients." These statements were also troublesome. The virus could transmit in its pre-symptomatic phase, or even asymptomatically, a phenomenon that was described in China. An outbreak soon gripped

Maui Memorial, and controversy engulfed the hospital when staff complained they were not informed of the cluster and were prohibited from wearing their own PPE when supplies ran short.

On March 6, Hawai'i encountered its first local case, a resident who became infected on the *Grand Princess* cruise ship. Despite an absence of testing, Governor David Ige reassured the public that he didn't think there was any community spread in Hawai'i. Health officials emphasized that the patient lacked symptoms during his air travel back to the Islands, stating that there was "no risk" to other passengers on the plane. Lt. Gov. Josh Green, an emergency room doctor, expressed his concern: "I personally feel if cruise ships are going to continue they have to be empowered to test people on the cruise ships. They should take a very hard look at whether or not they should hit the pause button for ninety days." But Park sounded a different tone, saying there's "no reason for us to track anyone" and "scare people unnecessarily."

On March 8, local media reported that only seventeen tests for SARS-CoV-2 had been performed by the DOH. On March 10, the department announced their intention to randomly screen two-hundred influenza specimens per week. The surveillance screening was a reasonable step. But for several weeks in February and early March, the state imposed restrictions on testing based on patient under investigation (PUI) definitions from the CDC that relied, in part, on patient travel history. This meant that clinicians had trouble accessing tests. By late February, the travel requirements for testing were nonsensical, as infection was becoming widespread throughout the world.

On March 13, the DOH issued guidance for spring break activities. Bruce Anderson, the health director, reassured the public that he didn't want to ruin their plans; he did ask people to take precautions such as covering coughs and washing hands. The president of the University of Hawai'i echoed this advice on March 16: "The good news is that even as new COVID-19 cases have been confirmed in Hawai'i, none are yet connected to any UH campus and none yet appear to be the result of any community transmission within the state. *This can change at any time as testing increases across the islands* [emphasis added.]" In other words, officials were aware that the reason they weren't finding cases is because they weren't looking for them. But this didn't prompt deeper reflection. President David Lassner concluded his message by affirming that campuses would remain open.

In mid to late March, as the state began experiencing cases and then deaths, the tone became more sober. Warnings against gathering in crowds and unnecessary travel became more frequent. Event cancellations began to ramp up. Instead of reassurance, there were warnings. On March 17, Governor Ige suggested that residents avoid gathering in groups greater than ten. This was in line with updated federal guidelines from the CDC. The DOH belatedly conceded the gravity of the situation. "You should act as though you have COVID and everyone around you does, too," said Bruce Anderson on April 3. That was the unvarnished truth. But by then Hawai'i was in the grip of its first wave, and claiming "the risk is low" was no longer tenable. Despite their rhetorical adjustments, the Health Department's reluctance to test continued obdurately until Governor Ige jettisoned its leadership in September.

There was a notable exception to Hawai'i's torpid pandemic response, one that would stand in contrast to the state leadership in Honolulu. On March 2, the Kaua'i mayor, Derek Kawakami, issued a press release asking residents of that island to "get prepared," with a list of suggestions including preparing for school closures and stay-at-home requests. He followed with an emergency proclamation on March 4 that authorized the county government to begin proactive planning for pandemic-related disruption. Over subsequent days, the county issued multiple announcements and decisions aimed at curbing disease spread. This included closing recreational facilities (March 12), addressing concerns over water transmission (March 13), closing marketplaces (March 13), suspending police–community relations events (March 13), and transitioning all county government offices from in-person to remote activity (March 16).

On March 18, Kawakami announced a curfew from 9 p.m. through 5 a.m., and he spoke directly to the people of the island:

> After taking an assessment of what will likely be a very long journey for all

> of us and the amount of limited resources we have, specifically public safety, first responder, and healthcare workers, we must take **bold steps** to ensure that our public safety officials, first responders, and healthcare workers have the necessary environment in which to keep us all safe.

He went on to explain several emergency steps, including a ban on pleasure travel. "Until further notice, visitors should not be traveling to our island for recreational purposes. . . Kauaʻi is on vacation."

That final line became the motto for Kauaʻi residents who took pride in their island's struggle against the virus. There was no apologetic reassurance here, and it's notable that at such an early date Kawakami was explicit in his expectation that the crisis would persist indefinitely. This candor characterized his ongoing communications. As subsequent events showed, he consistently refused to fall into line with state policies that increased the risk of transmission on Kauaʻi. He was aided by the Kauaʻi district health officer, Janet Bereman, who showed a healthy independence from the DOH on Oʻahu.

It was in early March that I had my first unpleasant experience of the confusion brought on by the new pandemic. It started with a brief phone call to the Department of Health. I was already weary of the reassurance they provided at press conferences. But it was during this time, the eerie quiet before the storm, that I requested my first test for SARS-CoV-2. It was for a patient who began coughing during her hospital stay; she worked in the tourism industry. The DOH refused the test on the grounds that she didn't have a high-risk travel history. I pointed out that this was not a good reason to decline a test, as there were already three large epidemics happening outside China and numerous cases in other countries. But they stuck to their talking point.

In response, I put the patient on airborne isolation, and that's when the sobering reality of the situation struck me. As soon as I entered the order, the tension on the floor rose noticeably. Nurses and physicians, longtime colleagues, eyed me warily. I received a call from our own infection control officer and infectious diseases division chief, Erlaine

Bello. Testing resources were extremely limited, and as we couldn't test, there was no way of excluding the disease. This meant that once the isolation order took effect, there was no clear means of removing the patient from isolation. This created considerable anxiety. Bello visited the patient herself in order to assess the risk and reassure the staff.

As the antibiotic steward for the hospital from 2015 to 2019, I worked well with Bello on infection and antibiotic control problems. She had a reputation for being no-nonsense. In dealing with people outside the division, I was often the friendly face, but no one wanted to annoy Bello. We played this to our advantage in setting sensible policies governing antibiotic use, and our joint efforts were often successful. I considered us a team, and I knew that on the occasions I put my foot down, I would have her backing.

But I had left that job, and this was a different conversation. My decision to isolate the patient without a means to rule out the infection had put us both in an awkward position, one I hadn't considered in advance. We muddled through, and I sent the patient home with instructions not to go out or host guests.

Feeling a bit humbled by this experience, I attempted to clear the air with Bello:

> We don't have adequate community surveillance yet, so we can't say with any confidence what's here and what's not here. If the virus follows a similar pattern it has elsewhere, we may become aware of it through a healthcare facility problem. These people we admit every day who are flu negative and have COPD or some similar diagnosis are the ones that worry me, as are relatively "healthy" people with mild illness who are walking around in proximity to the sick ones...

My concerns about transmission in minimally symptomatic people proved all too reasonable. But Bello was in an impossible position due to the lack of testing capacity. She was doing her best with a bad hand. I had to learn in these early days how to stratify risk without access to tests, and this was my crash course. In the infectious diseases division, we needed some system of prioritizing the testing resource, and we needed to coordinate that as physicians. In subsequent cases, I contacted Bello directly, and we made isolation decisions together. As the hospital's private testing capacity increased, we were less reliant on the DOH, and she used the resource to protect patients and staff. Testing eventually became universal for admitted patients. But all of this was new and uncharted, and the toll of uncertainty caused strain, even amongst friends.

In the meantime, the Queen's pharmacy had—at my urging as well as others'– acquired a small supply of hydroxychloroquine. This was an old drug used for years to treat lupus patients. It has immune modulatory properties. Reports from China and Korea claimed success using chloroquine, a related but more toxic medicine, in treating SARS-CoV-2 patients. Those countries were writing guidelines that included these drugs in treatment protocols.

When our shipment arrived at Queen's, I felt a swell of satisfaction. I was agnostic on its utility and always assumed that clinical trials, already being done elsewhere, would clarify its role. But I also understood, as a clinician, that I needed to offer the patients something. At this point there was nothing to go on but small observational studies. For a family, though, hearing of the limitation of an observational study and then being offered no treatment often feels like abandonment.

Some of my colleagues disagreed and were comfortable, even resolved, to offer no medical treatment for an infection. I found it unlikely that our hospital in Hawai'i would determine the effectiveness of any treatment with a placebo-controlled trial, and I disliked the idea of withholding the treatment. There was precedent for using drugs under compassionate and emergency use protocols going back to the HIV epidemic. In fact, the National Institute of Health (NIH) infectious diseases chief, Anthony Fauci, pioneered that approach. As long as we followed the evolving evidence, practiced informed consent, and contributed what we could to the science, I was content to use off-label medicines to treat a new disease.

When I inquired about using the drug, however, the pharmacy demurred. A new hospital committee to deal with COVID-19 (as the disease was now being called), guided by our medicine chief, Scott Gallacher, determined the evolving strategy. This apparently included sequestering the supply of hydroxychloroquine for a placebo-controlled trial.

What a peculiar vision of the apocalypse this offered! Here was the pandemic bearing down on us, and we were in a perfect state of ignorance. Our DOH refused to offer tests on the grounds that Hawai'i had no cases, yet in a bit of perfectly circular logic, we couldn't find cases without testing. The medicine division withheld the hydroxychloroquine, while I groped for any treatment that could be found. I had been around Queen's long enough to be skeptical of new committees, and, while coming into alignment with Erlaine Bello on isolation matters, I sent the following grain of salt to Scott Gallacher:

> Would suggest including an ID person in any research discussions. Bello, myself, or Ben Thomas (who is likely the next ASP person) would be good options. You can choose whoever annoys you the least! But I'm concerned about a couple pitfalls here. One is doing a "me too" study comparing something to nothing. Nothing is likely to be unacceptable soon, with a bunch of research coming out the next few weeks and evolving practice guidelines at a number of institutions. Another pitfall is making the medication inaccessible. Ideally stewardship has some input here but can get it to the right people quickly and assist with relevant documentation... If you need help with a task that's in my wheelhouse please just ask.

At the time, I worried that the stewardship program, which I had led for five years, was now sidelined and without formal leadership.

Gallacher's intentions, though, were good, and Queen's soon worked these problems out. Bello and Gallacher came to a helpful arrangement, and two additional infectious diseases physicians (myself included) were invited to join a new medication advisory group to deal with COVID. One of the pharmacists invited was Lynn Matsukawa, who was my principal colleague from the stewardship program.

The new group, which Gallacher assisted but also allowed a wide breadth and independence, guided a number of clinical trials and treatment protocols long after hydroxychloroquine failed as a first-line treatment. I gained a better understanding of the research considerations represented by Todd Seto, who efficiently oversaw numerous protocols. Seto answered the objection of doing a me-too protocol on hydroxychloroquine by combining the Queen's trial data with that collected at other centers, allowing the local experience of the drug to contribute to the general knowledge. This assuaged my primary concern with a placebo-controlled study. But more importantly, the friendly arguments that played out between internists, critical care doctors, infectious disease specialists, pharmacists, and research scientists ensured that every medication decision was a thoughtful one. It took us some time to arrive at this happy state, but the benefits of open discussion grew and were obvious to all. I could ask for no more.

The month of February ended with a final trip to Waimea, on the Big Island, where I had a growing panel of patients at North Hawai'i Community Hospital. I always enjoyed rural healthcare. I had spent a month on Moloka'i during my third year of residency to get a taste of rural primary care. Queen's merged with North Hawai'i in 2016, and adding clinical services to neighboring islands was a long-term project. I enjoyed the monthly trips to Waimea; rather than rushing back to the city, I often stayed the night and listened to music, or took a walk down the main street in town. A favorite tune from these visits was "Waimea Cowboy," in which the singer croons that contrary to popular belief, the best cowboys are Hawaiian cowboys. The self-confidence of the town charmed me, as did the slower pace. My wife and I bought a small farmhouse in the nearby countryside, and after ten years of work in the city, we often talked of shifting my practice off O'ahu.

The return trip home, though, felt unsafe. Passengers were crowded into lines and then herded onto the plane. No one wore masks yet. I was acutely aware of the Hawai'i visitor numbers and the inability to test people. A few people coughed and we all breathed the same air. Denial, I realized, was a profound, likely an evolved, behavior. And yet soon chaos would be upon us, and this mundane picture of a crowd boarding an airplane would be viewed as an irresponsible precursor to disaster. Even worse, I was returning home to a darkening scene, one in which—by my own desire to extricate myself from Queen's administrative duties—I had been left without a formal role. I felt isolated at precisely the moment the storm would hit.

These made for unpleasant travel thoughts, and it was with a sense of my own smallness that I passed the flight gazing down at the mountains of the archipelago. ☙

Chapter Four

THE EPIDEMIC STRIKES

APRIL 30, 2020

606

HAWAIʻI

1,003,974	3,089,733
UNITED STATES	WORLD

COVID-19 cases (data sources: World Health Organization and Hawaii Department of Health)

It was physicians in Sacramento who burned off America's fog of denial. The doctors at UC Davis accepted a transfer on February 19 after colleagues at a smaller facility intubated the patient for respiratory failure. The UC doctors suspected COVID-19 and tried to obtain a test, despite the patient's lack of travel history. In a subsequent description of the scene, they alluded to their frustration:

> We requested COVID-19 testing by the CDC, since neither Sacramento County nor CDPH is doing testing for coronavirus at this time. Since the patient did not fit the existing CDC criteria for COVID-19, a test was not immediately administered. UC Davis Health does not control the testing process.

Given their concerns, the UC Davis team kept the patient isolated. On February 23, the CDC relented, and three days later doctors received the positive result. As the patient had no travel history, it was apparent that there was a brisk transmission chain in Northern California. This made national headlines, and the travel restrictions on testing began to loosen.

It's hard to overstate how much this policy of restricting testing based on travel history cost the United States during the critical month of February. Given the spread of the virus, the geographic criteria were irrelevant before they were even published. This was discernible given the reported cases outside China. Officials simply chose not to acknowledge it. Within a few weeks, sizable outbreaks were uncovered in California, Washington, and New York City. Analysis of the virus genotypes, using a method of counting mutations (a kind of biological clock), revealed that in some locations the virus had been circulating undetected for weeks. Not only had the virus reached the United States, but containment had already failed.

The first wave of COVID on the mainland United States was a national humiliation. In Washington, ICUs began filling up with patients, many infected at local nursing homes. Unlike their counterparts in Wuhan, China, American doctors and nurses were critically short of protective supplies like gowns and N95 masks. This was because many of the supply chains for medical equipment had been outsourced to China, and there was now an international rush on equipment. American business, which had long abandoned domestic manufacturing, had to resurrect it in a matter of weeks. This was a big lift, and social media soon flooded with images of medical transport personnel in makeshift gowns and inadequate masks. In contrast, the Chinese had powered air-purifying respirator (PAPR) suits.

A flurry of impromptu clinical advice characterized this chaotic period, as American doctors on the West Coast began to wrestle directly with the virus. In a March 8 post titled "Note from the front lines," Martha Blum, an infectious diseases doctor in Monterey, California, summarized the clinical syndrome:

> The most common presentation was one week prodrome of myalgias, malaise,

> cough, low grade fevers gradually leading to more severe trouble breathing in the second week of illness. It is an average of 8 days to development of dyspnea and 9 days to onset of pneumonia/pneumonitis. It is not like Influenza, which has a classically sudden onset. Fever was not very prominent in several cases.

She went on to describe the common laboratory findings, including low lymphocyte counts, as well as the most common radiographic finding. This was an infiltrate in the periphery of the lung, with the quality of ground glass, an unusual pattern of pneumonia that characterized COVID-19. Recognizing there was little time for peer-reviewed research, and that testing was still severely limited, such information proved invaluable, as did the published reports from Wuhan. Doctors shared advice on clinical management, PPE use, testing, and how to deal with exposures in the hospital. This pace of information sharing was unprecedented, and I often stayed up late reading these accounts and formulating my own ideas on how to recognize and treat the disease.

New York took the biggest hit. In late February it became apparent to disease surveillance specialists that there was a rise in influenza-like illness (known in the trade as ILI). The ILI network is a syndromic epidemiology tool designed to monitor seasonal influenza activity, and its beauty is that it's built around the low-tech method of counting people who complain of respiratory ailments. But now ILI wasn't tracking influenza, because flu cases were declining. The ILI spike was something new, and what it showed was a wave building in the New York area.

I remember reading a news item about the ILI surge just before the hospitals took the heavy blow. It was an elegant but brutal illustration of the predictive power of that tool. But as in Washington, DC, state and city leadership was slow to absorb the significance of the data, and it was soon too late to alter the course of events. The ILI surge in New York began to diverge from influenza in late February. On March 2, New York Mayor Bill de Blasio tweeted, "I'm encouraging New Yorkers to go on with your lives—get out on the town despite Coronavirus." He followed

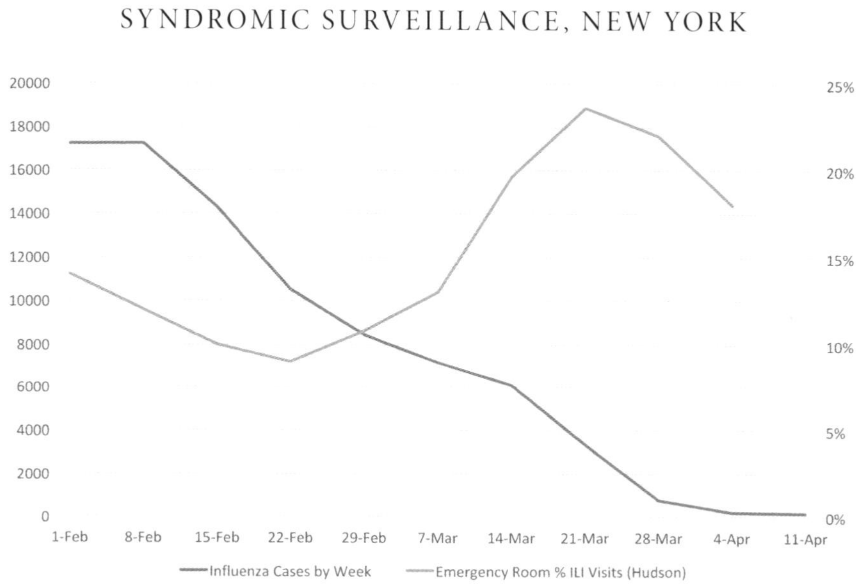

Figure 4.1 Data Source—New York Department of Health. Graph by author.

with a movie recommendation. On March 3, the media reported the first community transmission in the state. By March 18, New York had over three thousand confirmed cases. Governor Andrew Cuomo, finally recognizing the scale of events, locked the state down on March 20. This was two days—and thousands of cases—after Mayor Kawakami's announcement that "Kaua'i is on vacation."

The disease inundated hospitals in the most densely populated parts of the city, especially in the borough of Queens, and soon the ICUs filled and hospital workers became sick. Elmhurst Hospital, where I spent much of my fourth year of medical school, became ground zero for the New York epidemic. The surrounding community is one of the most diverse immigrant populations in the country, and crowded living arrangements are the norm. Many residents rely on public transport to get to blue-collar jobs all over the city. This community didn't stand a chance against a contagious respiratory virus.

Making matters worse, on March 25, the New York Department

of Health mandated that nursing homes receive COVID-19 infected patients. The order read:

> No resident shall be denied re-admission or admission to the NH solely based on a confirmed or suspected diagnosis of COVID-19. NHs are prohibited from requiring a hospitalized resident who is determined medically stable to be tested for COVID-19 prior to admission or re-admission.

The New York governor, Andrew Cuomo, later tried to justify this by arguing that New York was following federal policy. But the federal policy, dated March 13, said, "Nursing homes should admit any individuals that they would normally admit to their facility, including individuals from hospitals where a case of COVID-19 was/is present." That's not the same thing, and it is routine practice for nursing facilities to decline to accept transfer of patients diagnosed with a contagious disease.

Even if the federal authorities had mandated transfers of contagious patients to nursing homes, any sensible public health official would have refused such an order. This was a policy likely intended to assuage the bed control concerns of hospitals, but so lacking in infection control sense that it guaranteed a far deadlier outbreak.

The scale of death in New York's nursing homes wouldn't be fully appreciated for almost a year, due to a separate Cuomo scandal. By May 2020, there were reports of "at least 5,700" deaths in New York nursing homes, a large contributor to New York's total mortality figure. But the true number was closer to thirteen thousand deaths, and it was fifteen thousand including patients in assisted living and other forms of adult care. That figure didn't become apparent until late January 2021. That's when the state attorney general's office reported that the New York DOH failed to disclose thousands of deaths of nursing home residents who died after being transferred to local hospitals.

The upward revision in nursing home deaths came after the New York DOH ignored attempts by the state legislature to provide an accurate count of fatalities. New York officials stonewalled legislators on the death count out of fear that admission to the scale of the disaster would provide political ammunition to Republicans, who had requested the same information through the Justice Department. Cuomo's aide

Melissa DeRosa, while tossing a word salad, offered the state legislature the following explanation:

> [W]e were in a position where we weren't sure if what we were going to give to the Department of Justice, or what we give to you guys, what we start saying, was going to be used against us while we weren't sure if there was going to be an investigation.... That played a very large role in this.... [W]e do apologize. I do understand the position that you were put in. I know that it is not fair. It was not our intention to put you in that political position with the Republicans.

But there was no apology to the families of people who died. When New York assemblyman Ron Kim, a Democrat, criticized the Cuomo administration, he received a personal call from the governor. "We're in this business together and we don't cross certain lines, and he said I hadn't seen his wrath and that he can destroy me," said Kim, who subsequently hired a lawyer to serve as his intermediary with the Cuomo administration.

The poor handling of nursing homes in New York is a mistake that shines through the fog of the early COVID battlefield. It crystalizes in near-perfect resolution the groupthink of pre-pandemic American healthcare. And it stands as a warning to any doctor obsequious enough to betray their duty to patients on behalf of healthcare "administration."

The mortality rate during this first wave was high, and nowhere was it higher than New York. By mid-April there were ten thousand dead in the state, more than three times as many deaths as occurred during the September 11 attacks. I estimated the infection fatality rate at 1 percent, about ten times higher than seasonal flu. The situation was so bad that in some nursing homes, staff stopped coming to work. In one facility in neighboring New Jersey, police received an anonymous tip leading them to bodies. This was a vision of hell.

One of the worst aspects of the COVID-19 epidemic in New York was the way people died in isolation. With no intrinsic immunity to the disease, healthcare workers had to suit up for each patient encounter, and hospitals restricted their visitor policies to keep potentially infected family members off the treatment floors. Thousands of people died in isolation rooms, accompanied only by the chirps of IV pumps and telemetry machines.

New York's feuding city and state governments eventually settled on a policy of complete lockdown. The experience of Italy thus repeated itself in the United States, but with one important difference. In the United States there was no federal leadership, and each state charted its own course. Smaller epidemics in other parts of the country, several of which appeared to be seeded directly from New York, based on genetic analysis of the circulating variants, were met with far less vigorous shutdowns. And so while the epidemic in New York abated in May, it quietly spread to other states. And while Italy and other European countries saw their epidemics fall off, the US entered a dangerous plateau of about twenty thousand cases per day. This presaged further disaster, though with the

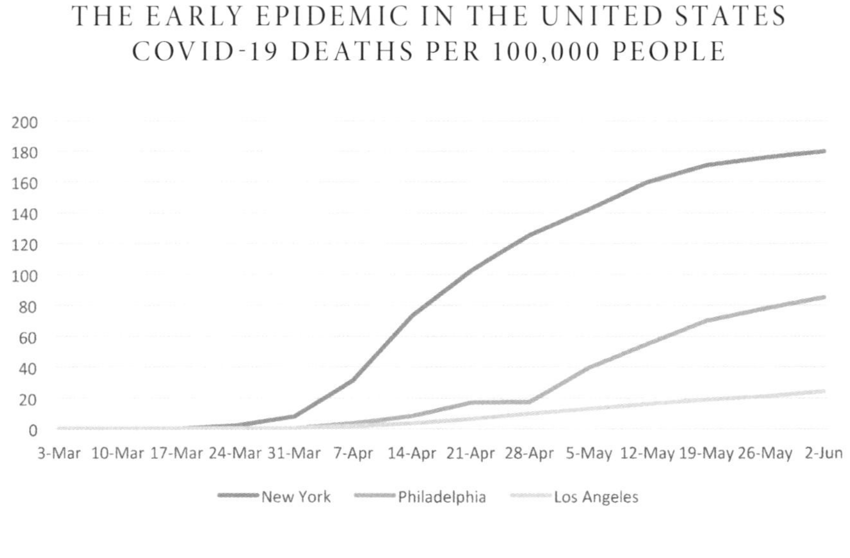

Figure 4.2 Data Source—USA Facts, CDC. Graph by author.

weather warming in the late spring, many downplayed the possibility.

The scale of death in New York in the spring did not prevent a tsunami of sanctimony and self-congratulation from its government and their boosters in the media. Andrew Cuomo received fawning press coverage, particularly on CNN, where despite conflict of interest rules, his brother, Chris Cuomo, covered him. In a media environment obsessed with Trump, Cuomo's confrontation with the president formed a telegenic part of the melodrama. He was portrayed, in the words of Billy Crystal, as "the epitome of New York tough." Somehow in the midst of all this manliness, and despite the mortality crisis consuming his state, Cuomo found time to write a best-selling book, on leadership no less. And in a delicious bit of irony, the International Academy of Television Arts and Sciences awarded him an Emmy "in recognition of his leadership during the Covid-19 pandemic and his masterful use of television to inform and calm people around the world." The accompanying celebrity salutes, which aged like flat champagne, made for useful grist on right wing media.

Watching this from Hawaiʻi, I couldn't understand what New Yorkers had to feel good about. Even before the extent of the Cuomo scandals became apparent, a brief look at the death figures made it clear that New York's pandemic response was a wreck. I assumed Trump was useless, as did all my colleagues. It was Cuomo and de Blasio I worried the state would imitate. My firmest desire in April and May of 2020 was that Hawaiʻi not follow the path of New York. For those paying attention to the epidemic, as opposed to the media narrative, New York's government was the epitome of failure.

Why are hypocrisy and false narrative so toxic to a public health response? Why do I harp on them in New York and other places, when Trump's failures were so much larger in scale? Because success in a pandemic requires social cohesion, trust in authorities, and shared sacrifice. Dishonesty, even when it seems benign, and especially when it's convenient for one side's political purposes, is the weed that chokes these virtues.

Looking back on the entrance of SARS-CoV-2 into the United States, the overwhelming impression is that of a sustained lack of candor from public officials. This was relentless dishonesty, and it was bipartisan. It may have been the only area of public life that everyone agreed on. Americans had vastly different ideologies in the spring of 2020, but a willingness to be BSed by people who told them what they wanted to hear was the vice they held in common. ♈

Chapter Five

BATTEN DOWN THE HATCHES

My concern that the country would soon experience a major disruption related to the pandemic took on magnified significance as New York's hospitals spiraled into chaos. Not having administrative responsibilities at the hospital afforded me time to engage a wider group of people outside of Queen's. James Ireland, soon to become a critical figure in the lieutenant governor's team, invited me to join their weekly calls.

It was during one of these calls that David Derauf entered my scene. Energetic and dissatisfied, he wanted to know every kind of detail in the state's response. What was the testing capacity on Oʻahu? What were they doing to mitigate the risk to public housing, which was the densest in the state?

These were trenchant questions, and David asked them with an urgency that no one else possessed. I spotted a kindred spirit, and I contacted him separately after a call. This was the beginning of my most fruitful partnership during the pandemic. From that point on, David and I were an inseparable pair, each supporting the other's efforts, each merging our distinct clinical perch into a greater whole.

David Derauf is an internist with a public health degree. He's originally from Minnesota, but for three decades he has been the director of Kōkua Kalihi Valley. This is one of the major primary care health centers in town, providing service to Kalihi Valley, the most densely urban part of Honolulu. His patient population includes much of the Pacific Islander community and thousands of people who live in public housing. This group overlapped considerably with the population I cared for at Queen's. His organization, known as KKV, has a reputation for doing innovative work, including mobilizing hundreds of clinic patients to grow their own food through a large community garden.

I first met David when I was a resident at University of Hawaiʻi Internal Medicine Residency Program (UHIMRP). But I became subsumed in my clinical duties and didn't keep in touch. I recognized him quickly on the lieutenant governor's call. He has a distinct, wiry energy, like a spring under great tension. He's thin with a face that is younger by at least a decade than his actual age. He's often the smartest person in the room, and he reads constantly. My e-mail in-box was soon full of articles. These became a deluge that I could barely keep up with, and my own rate of return fire was more modest. In conversation, David betrays his Minnesota roots. There's a directness that borders on irritability and a presumption (sometimes incorrect) that everyone else wants to do the right thing. He becomes frustrated with anyone who obfuscates, but he is also bighearted and humorous. I could make him laugh, often by jabbing at our interactions with officialdom. We found companionship in crisis, and I made a new friend.

In March, the hospital began to see COVID-19. One morning, a colleague in the radiology department wanted to show me something. He pulled up a CT chest scan from a patient in the emergency room. There was a hazy infiltrate, like ground glass, that spared the center of the lungs while filling the peripheral edges. This I recognized from the online clinical threads, and from the medical literature from China. "Where's the patient?" I asked. Discharged home. The DOH had declined to test.

The tension at Queen's was becoming extreme. I fired numerous e-mails to Chris Whelen, the micro lab director at Diagnostic Lab Services (DLS), urging him to develop an independent testing capacity:

> Now that the FDA has relaxed regulations and is allowing for lab developed tests, can we get a novel Coronavirus PCR available for clinicians?
>
> I realize there may be a temptation to do this all through DOH, but given the problems and delays they are having, it would be excellent to have our own option in the QMC/DLS system. As a clinician having people cough on you and not being able to rule out the worst pathogen is bad for morale, to put it mildly.

The response I received was that the lab couldn't move until testing and reporting was coordinated with the DOH. I thought the law should be no obstacle, and that any regulator who wanted to hamper physicians should take my dare. Whelen was under great strain at this time. He had a deep and symbiotic relationship with DOH. But he also understood the basic imperative to get the tests into the hands of the doctors. By late March, he had succeeded. DLS ran its own machine on island, a Roche, and could do hundreds of tests per week with a twenty-four-hour turnaround time. Queen's doctors no longer required approval from anyone in the state government. It was like the lights suddenly turned on, illuminating the field of play. Testing capacity continued to grow quickly, and the Queen's system soon ran thousands of tests per week with same-day turnaround.

This was just in time for the first wave. The sporadic cases of undiagnosed pneumonia were followed a couple weeks later by dozens of patients coming in with respiratory failure. The size of the iceberg was quickly becoming evident.

Eric Crawley, a critical care doctor at Straub, contacted me shortly after my Facebook post at the end of February. Eric was a mentor from residency. I remember doing an evening ICU call at Queen's with him, probably in 2008. ICU shifts, especially at night, are an exercise in extreme medicine. Procedures done are generally in an emergency, with high stakes. This isn't my thing, but amongst ICU doctors, Eric had the perfect personality for it. There was a touch of dark humor, a calmness in chaos, and he didn't take himself too seriously. It's not a coincidence that he's former military. Stoicism and a talent for triage run deep in the service.

Eric asked for my help with an organization the state was establishing to respond to the pandemic. This was the first time I heard of HI-EMA, the Hawai'i branch of the Federal Emergency Medical Agency (FEMA). Eric was assembling a team of people with different skills from amongst his contacts throughout the state. This included other colleagues of his from critical care and the medical school. He wanted me to offer advice on infectious diseases questions.

I agreed, and one of the first tasks he gave me was to model the potential impact of a wave of COVID-19 on the islands. I had never done modeling, but he didn't seem dissuaded by this. Though nervous, I was encouraged by this vote of confidence. I reviewed some of the prominent models that had been recently published, including those released by Imperial College in the UK and by the University of Washington in the United States. These had highly variable predictions of the size of the mortality event about to impact the United States. One thing that became clear to me was that the models were only as good as the assumptions plugged into them. This was later to be a big point of confusion, as people became angry when the models were "wrong." Having looked at them closely, I found these criticisms misdirected. The point of a model isn't to be "right"; it's to tell you what will happen under a given set of circumstances, so that you pull the correct lever and *change the circumstances*.

When I plugged in various assumptions for Hawai'i, using a University of Pennsylvania COVID modeling program, it became apparent that the exponential growth of the infection in the community would overwhelm any existing healthcare capacity in the state. I provided a couple of different projections, using different assumptions, to illustrate this point. Crawley had to report up a command chain, and ultimately HI-EMA was under a newly appointed general, Ken Hara. My message for Crawley and the general was simple. The rate of transmission was the critical variable, even more important than the mortality of the infection, because a brisk growth rate—multiplied exponentially—would translate into a much higher death count. I advised the general to maintain social discipline (in order to reduce transmission opportunities), and to go on offense by testing aggressively and establishing an effective quarantine system. I emphasized that they must wrap their heads around the notion of exponential growth, as this was a key difference between a human and viral enemy. "We can't vent our way out of this," I concluded.

Much of the early failure in public health messaging was due to a misunderstanding of risk, a result of confusion regarding exponential growth. If there are twenty cases of a virus in a large city, and the fatality rate is 1 percent, it's easy to tell people "the risk is low." But if those cases are doubling every three days, and the city fails to interrupt that growth, then in just a few weeks things begin to get out of hand. In about a month you are dealing with tens of thousands of cases and hundreds of deaths.

As the healthcare system becomes overwhelmed, doctors and nurses fall ill, and the fatality rate climbs well above 1 percent. Any conversation about risk that fails to take exponential growth into account doesn't make sense.

I didn't realize it at the time, but HI-EMA had access to professional modelers, including Tim Brown of the East-West Center. I met Tim during a trip to the Diamond Head command bunker where HI-EMA had established its operations. With a sturdy jaw and a patch over his right eye, Tim looked like he belonged in the command bunker. He spoke with a quiet intensity, and though polite, I could sense his dissatisfaction with the state's preparations. He gave a lucid talk with a detailed analysis of the various modeling paradigms. I asked a few questions and chased him down afterwards for a conversation. We stood outside, where it was hot and bright. Web-based meetings were not yet common, and I felt relieved to be out from the conference rooms. Here was a person who obviously had the intellectual chops to advise the state effort on epidemiology questions. I was relieved to find that Tim's conclusions, though better informed, largely matched my own.

General Hara did not attend Tim Brown's talk, and I doubt he ever read my memo. Comments he made later in the summer suggest that he struggled to grasp exponential growth. But it was that growth—not the deadliness of individual infections—that made the virus ferocious. This ability to replicate quickly and overwhelm a human response was the adaptation that made SARS-CoV-2 a terrible foe. Many officials in the state did not understand they were in an evolutionary knife fight. They lacked a sense of urgency in standing up systems that would tackle this most crucial variable. I felt sure that either we would be on offense against the virus, stamping out transmission chains wherever we could find them, or it would be on offense against us, crushing our hospitals and killing hundreds or even thousands of people.

My involvement with HI-EMA ended when Steve Hankins was put in charge of Emergency Support Function (ESF) #8, the medical response team. I suspect that Ireland and Crawley were also briefly considered for the role. Either would have made a fine choice.

Hankins had a background as the family practice director for the UH residency program. He told me that he had years of experience in public health, including in the FEMA response to Hurricane Katrina. I found it odd that he mentioned that episode. I had the sinking feeling that Hawaiʻi would soon be dealing with its own Katrina. Nonetheless they had asked for my help, and so I plowed ahead:

> Steve, Eric –
>
> This is just to follow up on yesterday evening's call. I would like to confirm that I am tasked with advising ESF-8 on matters pertaining to isolation and quarantine. I understand this does not confer authority to establish a quarantine. However I will use you (and the ESF-8 structure) as my reference point while engaging subject experts and community leaders on these topics.
>
> My initial goal will be to establish communication between stakeholders and help coordinate community efforts to arrange safe isolation for COVID patients. I will encourage acts of volunteerism from community stakeholders that hold the potential to reduce transmission. When assistance is requested (financial, logistical, etc.) that is beyond my scope, I will refer these issues up our command chain to you. I will keep you both in the loop with brief but regular updates.
>
> I hope this is acceptable, please let me know.

My apprehension was confirmed when Crawley told me that I would not be the point person on the quarantine problem. Instead, this function was turned over to the Department of Health, and I was to report to their representative. I was a bit surprised by this, as the evening before they had asked me to work on it. I had already contacted several fellow physicians to form a well of expertise that could advise the effort. Hankins didn't respond to my e-mail and left it for Crawley to deliver the blow. From that point forward, I was no longer invited to any HI-EMA strategy meetings.

Some people may have taken this personally, but I felt some relief. My clinical practice was a full-time job, and I soon had to wrestle directly with the virus. It was also increasingly clear that HI-EMA would not be effective, at least at the crucial task of controlling transmission.

A month later, during the peak of the first wave, I spoke once more with Hankins. He called me because I was making noise that the quarantine issue hadn't been fixed, and I wasn't able to safely discharge patients. It was a meandering conversation. I believe he made a genuine effort to be friendly towards me. But at one point he told me what he really thought of containment. He thought that shutting down the entire state was an error, and that he was focused on the big picture, which included the collateral damage of such a move. On quarantine he had little to say, deferring to the DOH and declining to help me with the problem.

This view, which Hankins expressed to me in private, was entirely consistent with statements he made in public. Speaking to University of Hawai'i News in May, he said:

> When we finally look back on this pandemic, we want to have reduced the overall illness and death in the state of Hawai'i related to all of the impacts of COVID-19—not just from the virus itself, but all of the health effects that come from the disruption of healthcare and other critical services. We must also mitigate the health-related consequences of the economic impacts across all of our sectors, short- and long-term.

I have no doubt Hankins believed this, and that his intentions were good. But the problem with zooming out to such a broad view is that it allows you to evade responsibility for particulars. There were actions that the state needed to take to reduce viral transmission. The state was not taking them. This would have a direct impact on the size of the mortality event. But the conversation was about "health-related consequences" across "all of our sectors."

This style of evasion—in which government uses generalities to avoid accountability for important details—reminded me of a Vaclav Havel essay I read during college. Writing in 1965 about two incidents when window ledges crumbled off poorly maintained buildings and killed pedestrians, Havel noted that the communist government had done nothing to fix the problem, but in the newspaper had waxed poetically about broader social progress in the country. Havel mocked this kind of talk and complimented people for seeing through it:

> As it had done many times before, the public again showed more intelligence

> and humanity than the writer, for it had understood that the so-called prospects of mankind are nothing but an empty platitude if they distract us from our particular worry about who may be killed by a third window ledge, and what will happen should it fall on a group of nursery school children out for a walk.

HI-EMA had no plan for stopping viral transmission, which was the crumbling window ledge above our heads. And the grand, sweeping view of healthcare in Hawaiʻi was, in early 2020, a distraction. The new virus was far more deadly than influenza, and the lack of immunity meant it could spread more aggressively through the population. A scenario of uncontrolled transmission would stifle the economy as people became ill and businesses shut down. An island full of multigenerational homes had little chance of separating the elderly from infected young people. And economic data from around the world was soon to show that preventing transmission was a prerequisite to navigating the economic fallout. In fact, that would become the basis of the successful tier system that Honolulu eventually settled on.

This disagreement reflected a broader dispute over the role of public health in responding to the pandemic. Influenced by the success of countries like Korea, David Derauf and I advocated a vigorous system of test-trace-isolate. This triad, which later expanded to become test-trace-isolate-support, was the cornerstone of the containment strategy. Aggressive and targeted use of testing would allow the state to identify where transmission was happening. Not testing, in my view, was analogous to boxing with a blindfold. But for the testing to be useful, it had to be combined with contact tracing, so that all contacts of identified cases were also tested and placed in quarantine. And each identified case must be isolated from friends and family while contagious, and supported through that interval.

Yet in many states, and in many countries, test-trace-isolate failed. Given that a lot of transmission occurred amongst asymptomatic or pre-symptomatic patients, it was difficult to get the upper hand on the virus using these tools. As systems became overwhelmed, keeping up with thousands of cases became impossible. There was a legitimate argument to be had over the role of test-trace-isolate in the disease response strategy, especially in states like New York that already had widespread transmission. But the failure to contain the epidemic using public health tools led to lockdowns that were damaging economically and socially. The best way to avoid collateral damage was to succeed at public health.

I thought it defeatist, and disqualifying, for public officials to abandon containment strategies in Hawaiʻi. Test-trace-isolate had just succeeded in countries in Asia and the Pacific, some with much larger populations than Hawaiʻi. Hawaiʻi had control over its border, by sea and by air, and the state possessed excess hotel capacity that could be used to support an entry quarantine. Federal money was soon to become available to support a range of public health initiatives. The state had small companies led by dynamic entrepreneurs who were interested in developing everything from contact tracing software to locally manufactured rapid antigen tests. Most importantly, Hawaiʻi didn't yet have widespread transmission, or anything close to it. There was no reason to despair. I felt that if we did not strain every nerve to keep the disease out, we would be derelict in our duty.

Not everyone agreed with my bleak view of HI-EMA, and some who agreed remained inside the tent. Eric Crawley soldiered on, and as he had responsibility for the critical care piece, he made contributions in boosting the state's readiness with ICU and ventilator capacity. HI-EMA also performed a valuable function in receiving and distributing medicines. In this mitigative role they showed greater comfort, as it did not require breaking down bureaucratic turf or fighting with the DOH. General Hara supported the use of the military for contact tracing, a critical component of transmission control, although due to DOH resistance, that resource was deployed too late to be as impactful as it should have been.

Though unsuccessful, my efforts to form a team for Crawley were not wasted. I was soon in contact not just with David Derauf, but with several other gifted individuals. Tim Brown joined our conversations, and he added value through his ability to rapidly digest epidemiologic data and generate his own models. Chad Meyer, a tropical medicine doctor on Maui with years of experience in public health through prior work for the State Department, contributed to our discussions. I also met Jerry Murphy, a military infectious diseases doctor at Tripler. He worked well with Steve Hankins and was later invited into the HI-EMA deliberations.

By now, none of us were under illusions that the state's public health response to the early epidemic would be a robust one. Though he had replaced me in the HI-EMA tent, I liked Jerry. He was passionate about doing his duty to protect the state, and he brought a Navy man's discipline to the task. I thought he must be a far more patient person than me to sit through their meetings and maintain good cheer. He became a friendly voice inside the state response.

It's odd that at this time I didn't lose heart. Looking back, there was little to inspire confidence. But I never doubted Hawaiʻi could win. I felt I had spent my whole life preparing for this test. The circumstances beyond my control only elevated my sense of purpose. To grapple with the beast, and help drive it from the Islands, was a duty I felt bound to. I was heartened by the number of brilliant people with whom I had recently become acquainted. I felt a camaraderie towards them that soon dwarfed my disappointments. I was sure that as a group, scientists and physicians possessed more talent and moral authority than the people occupying political positions, and that, grinning through these early defeats, we would ultimately prevail. This was my mood as David Derauf and I began the work of building our own band of experts to fight the disease.

Chapter Six

THE WITCHING TIME

'Tis now the very witching time of night,
When churchyards yawn, and hell itself breathes out
Contagion to this world.
–*HAMLET*, ACT III, SCENE 2

The witching time was upon us, and the long night of COVID-19 would last for many months. I remember a Sunday, my last day off before the first surge of sick patients. My family took a trip to Waimānalo. I sat listlessly, staring out the window as we passed Koko Head. Surf broke against rocks, and sea foam mixed with air as the car turned around the coast. I was quiet, gazing on the scenery, but my heart beat fast in my chest. A peculiar sensation filled me, like breathing in cold, dry air. I realized this was fear, and I had never felt it before at the hospital. That itself was an amusing observation. I had taken care of countless patients with tuberculosis, *Staph aureus*, and viral pathogens like HIV and hepatitis. Once during residency, doing a procedure late at night, I had stuck myself with a needle. That required a battery of follow-up tests to ensure I wasn't infected. At other times, I cared for patients who were aggressive because they were withdrawing, psychotic, or drunk. But at no point during any of those experiences was I afraid.

Now I was. I thought of the doctor who died in China, and of dead doctors and nurses on the Mainland. I thought of our equipment shortages and our problems testing people. I was about to meet the virus, and the virus was on offense. The state expected casualties. No one would blink if I was one of them.

When we reached Waimānalo, I peeled off from my family. I sprinted down the beach a couple hundred yards until I was exhausted. I lay in the sand, gasping for air, my eyes fixed on sunbeams passing through the clouds. The light seemed to be carrying something; it was tiny, speckled, and multitudinous. I imagined the virus itself visiting me through the sky, bathing me in this strange light. This was the world now, grotesque and deadly.

Then the daydream lifted. I caught my breath. The light appeared normal, and the sky was again azure. I thought I might die in the next few weeks, but that this would be a good way for it to happen—in the service of friends and neighbors.

With that notion taking root, I was relieved to find that my mind had banished fear.

There's no doubt that waiting for SARS-CoV-2 was, for me, much worse than SARS-CoV-2. I suffered through weeks in February and March, when we were hampered by poor testing resources, worried that I would miss a case and be responsible for seeding an outbreak in the hospital. But when the virus hit, it wasn't subtle. Over a period of about a week, Queen's admitted a dozen patients with respiratory failure. The clinical presentations were variable, but most had cough, fever, shortness of breath, and low oxygen saturation. The chest x-rays showed the typical peripheral pneumonia, but with testing available, doctors stopped using the CT scanner to help with diagnosis. Any transportation of patients through the hospital increased the risk of transmission.

The patients were different ages, and I had a fair number who were young or middle age. The notion that the disease only impacts the elderly, by then part of the narrative spreading on the internet, was untrue for my patients. The first confirmed case I had was a young woman in her twenties who had severe pneumonia and briefly went to the ICU. That said, the young tended to recover, and the elderly did worse.

This was one important difference between SARS-CoV-2 and the influenza virus that struck America in 1918. That virus had been particularly brutal to young people, and the highest mortality rates were amongst people twenty to thirty years old. In 1918, influenza ravaged military barracks, in some encampments leaving hundreds dead. When SARS-CoV-2 visited the military in 2020, it raced through the population with similar speed, but only a few young people died. In 1918, thousands of families were destroyed as children became orphans. If there was one mercy to SARS-CoV-2, it was the tendency to spare the young. But the notion that it only sickened the elderly was false. Queen's would care for hundreds of young and middle-aged adults who arrived short of breath and hypoxic, and in the absence of supportive medical care like oxygen therapy, many more would have died.

The hospital transformed itself in April. No visitors were allowed. Elective surgeries were canceled. The food court was closed except for takeout. Security kiosks were established at every entrance to check IDs and measure temperatures. Tower 9 Diamond Head, usually designated for a mix of medical and surgical patients, became the COVID unit. The sicker patients went to the medical intensive care unit (MICU) on Tower 4. At the peak of the first wave, Queen's filled Tower 9 with confirmed cases and rule outs, and about half the MICU was also COVID.

The COVID floors had a sparse aesthetic. Like battleships that had cleared their decks, all superfluous equipment and personal belongings were removed. The entrance doors were closed, and warning signs were posted. Around the unit, each patient's room had additional signage warning people to stay out or instructing them on how to don and doff equipment. N95 masks were in such short supply that these were kept in the nurse manager's room. To get one, I had to state my purpose, and after using it, I put it in a brown paper bag with my name attached. These were then sterilized with ultraviolet light and reused. Along the hallways, face shields, each individually assigned, hung from pegs in the walls. The ward reminded me of a favorite movie from childhood, when a deck of the starship *Enterprise* was taken over by the Borg.

I was fighting an alien, and with the dreadful waiting over, I felt exhilaration and relief. Each day I drove to work and blasted music at high volume. A favorite song at this time was "Bullet In A Gun," which I had pilfered from my preteen's music list. It was loud and poppy, nothing like my usual tastes, but it was also fatalistic, and it suited the mood. I drove above the speed limit on the now empty freeway. Hyper-caffeinated and high on purpose, I wondered if this was what cocaine felt like.

Prior to the hospital initiating its N95 recycling practice, the supply was so short that I started carrying construction N95s in my back pocket.

These were donated from friends and relatives who had used them to remodel garages and do other housework. I didn't want to take a medical N95 when I was in and out of a room in ten minutes, while a nurse had to work a shift all day. I used the construction masks and rotated between them every five days or so. When the hospital began UV recycling, I adjusted course. I preferred the regular medical N95, nuked, to the construction masks. The data to support N95 recycling at that time was not good, but neither was the data for anything else I was doing.

I thought it likely I would get sick, and I set up an area in the basement of my home where I could rest. Each day when I returned home, I scrubbed down in the outside shower, then relaxed in my room. The concrete floor was cool, and I stretched out on a makeshift bed. Around me were pictures of family who had passed, as well as those of old friends. I hung a few mementos from my youth: a wine skin from Spain, a flag I had brought home from Kurdistan, a *hamsa* for good luck. When bananas fruited in my yard, I cut them down with a machete and strung the stalk from the ceiling. The bananas spun slowly as breeze passed through the windows, sap dripping on newspaper on the floor. It was a pleasant room for a nap, a bohemian refuge in the tropics.

I inquired about a hotel room but soon realized that quarantine for healthcare workers, like everyone else, had been fumbled. I tried to send my family to the Big Island so I could avoid the risk of infecting them, but Layla objected. We were in it together. And in the end, Layla and the kids were not fond of my attempts to self-isolate. It became obvious that whenever I got sick, they would get sick. Many doctors and nurses were in the same situation, and my disgust with the failure to procure protective gear and quarantine facilities deepened into a kind of personal dislike of the authorities. But I also understood that this was an occupational hazard, and after choosing a career in infectious diseases, I had no intention of passing the pandemic in my basement, cozy as it was.

The Queen's infectious diseases division was a group of individualists who liked to set their own schedules. For weekend coverage, we were organized into two on-call teams to cover Queen's and other hospitals in town. This worked well enough for ordinary illnesses, but for COVID it made no sense. I didn't want to round on COVID patients and then visit the oncology floor to examine people getting chemotherapy. It was time for a division of labor with some central direction.

After discussions with Erlaine Bello, who continued as the infectious diseases chief, the division settled on a COVID call schedule, and I took the first two weeks at Queen's in early April. As the on-call infectious diseases doctor for COVID, I interacted with the medical ICU doctors and the general internists. These were the two services caring for COVID patients at Queen's. I spoke with the Health Department about patient disposition. My goal was to ensure that any patient I saw did not transmit the infection to another person. I spoke at length with families, educating them in infection control and arranging any needed follow-up. The division had two doctors on at any given time, and I worked with Jamie Joyner and Ben Thomas. Both were excellent, and in sharing the burden, we reduced the variability between our practices.

There were a few common clinical questions people asked me during infectious diseases consultations in this early phase. The most basic related to diagnosis. Early on, we couldn't test, so the question essentially amounted to "how worried should I be, and what level of isolation should the patient be on?" Later, the questions involved interpretation of test results. People were concerned about false negative results in patients who clinically acted like COVID, discrepant results from different testing platforms, or false positive results in patients who were improving but kept testing positive.

One patient from the first wave made a particular impression. The patient had a glaring, travel-related risk factor for acquiring SARS-CoV-2, and both the symptoms and radiographic findings suggested COVID pneumonia. But the test was negative, and two separate repeats also came back negative. After a couple weeks spinning my wheels, my partner, Joe Koo, texted me irritably. He suggested I go down a different route, and soon afterwards I diagnosed HIV and an opportunistic pneumonia. This was humbling for me, because under ordinary circumstances I would have made that diagnosis quickly. I allowed myself to be blinded by adrenaline and the emotion of the moment. Fortunately, the patient recovered on the correct treatment, and my pride was the primary victim. But as was often the case, my senior partner made me a better doctor. In subsequent months, I would filter out the noise of pandemic anxieties, and I diagnosed a few patients with alternative syndromes (including some that were noninfectious) that appeared, on admission, to be COVID.

Another common question pertained to hydroxychloroquine, which at that time was the only available treatment. On this issue I interfaced with the critical care group and Todd Seto's clinical trials team. Queen's had a trial where patients were randomized to drug or placebo. Through the medical advisory group, the hospital also had an off-label use indication, which meant that doctors could offer it outside the context of the clinical trial. This was a compromise between people with differing opinions, and it was consistent with guidelines at larger institutions. Many patients just wanted the drug, and so the off-label indication came at the expense of the clinical trial. My own experiences with it were mixed. I treated the young woman with it, and she rapidly improved. Some of my colleagues thought this was a good success, but she was healthy and young. I suspect I could have run her over with a moped, and she would have gotten better. Older patients on the drug got worse. My overall impression was that it probably did nothing, and that's what the clinical trial data later showed.

The last question was the most important from a public health perspective, and that was disposition of infected patients. In April, it wasn't yet clear how long patients were contagious. I knew from the literature published by Chinese doctors that many patients remained positive in their molecular test for weeks, but most patients experienced resolution of symptoms within seven to ten days. Did the persistent positive test mean the patient was contagious, or did it just indicate fragments of viral RNA? As more data came in, the latter explanation proved to be most common. But with imperfect information to guide me, I insisted on no discharge of any patient who continued to test positive back into a crowded housing situation. If they couldn't have their own bedroom and bathroom at home, I blocked the discharge and requested a hotel room. This created a bit of a stir, but I thought it important to hold the line on disease transmission during discharge planning. Most of my colleagues agreed with me, and the hospital began working on its own hotel arrangements with local businesses. I was pleased to see the Queen's administration take such an enlightened view of the matter, and it helped inform later efforts at the city and state level.

On March 16, Honolulu mayor Kirk Caldwell announced he would cancel all events on city property. This included the convention center. He followed this on March 23 with another emergency order instructing all Oʻahu residents to stay at home and work from home. Schools were closed, and businesses shuttered. This prompted the governor, David Ige, to announce a statewide lockdown starting on March 25. On March 21, the governor also imposed a fourteen-day quarantine on all passengers arriving from outside Hawaiʻi, and this was extended to interisland travel on April 1.

Collectively, these moves were the most impactful actions taken by local and state government in Hawaiʻi. Over a period of just a couple weeks, the authorities had gone from reassuring the public to closing down every communal activity. Life came to a sudden and jarring halt. Tourism plummeted by more than 90 percent, and people who came and violated quarantine were subject to arrest. This was similar to the reaction of governments in New York and California, but Hawaiʻi benefited from being an island state and earlier in its epidemic curve.

Most of my cases were travel-related, and a number of my patients had recently returned from Las Vegas or were family members of travelers who did. I was convinced that the early epidemic on Oʻahu was the Las Vegas epidemic. This suggested that Hawaiʻi largely dodged the bullet in February and March, with little or no introduction of virus from Asia and little community spread.

The lockdown crushed the epidemic curve, but it took a few weeks for me to feel that effect in the hospital. In the meantime, Tower 9 Diamond Head and the MICU continued to fill, and the wave peaked at fifteen to twenty admitted patients. It felt like a wave, too, one that built quickly and then receded just as fast. In retrospect, the peak number wasn't much, but to put it in perspective, I had never, in ten years, seen seasonal influenza fill half the MICU. By any sensible metric, this was a severe epidemic, logarithmically worse than seasonal flu, with the potential to overwhelm the hospital. I lost two patients, while a third developed a complication that left him sick for months.

The hospital medicine group had also built a COVID call schedule, and so I passed these early weeks with a rotating cast of internists. These were people I knew from prior infectious diseases and internal medicine work. The first week I was on with Ynhu Le. She was young, with a fresh face that smiled easily. She was also sharp and unflappable, despite the uncertainty threatening every clinical decision. She later joined the medication advisory group for the hospital, representing the frontline internists. After Ynhu Le's call week, Malia Ramirez and Ryan Honda took the helm. These two had years in leadership roles in the medicine division. When I showed up, now in my second week, looking tired and informal, I found them at the Tower 9 Diamond Head computer consoles. Well rested and dressed in freshly ironed scrubs, Ryan looked like a television actor. There was not a wrinkle in his clothing. Malia appeared as though she had traveled from beach to salon, and then onward to the hospital. Her hair tolerated not a single errant strand. Thin, tanned, and handsome, they looked fantastic. This was Hollywood in the Pacific. Never did two doctors arrive more smartly dressed for the viral apocalypse.

I let them have it, and there was some good-natured back and forth about end-of-world fashion. Maintaining sartorial standards throughout the week proved difficult. But they more than made up for it with thoughtful and compassionate clinical management. The mood was light despite the gloom around us. Towards the end of my second week, it was evident that the lockdown orders were working. When I handed my list over to my partner, Royden Young, the census had begun to dip. Within a few weeks, hospital services returned close to normal. By the time I was up again for COVID call, there was barely any COVID.

The first wave had receded as rapidly as it had risen. The death count in Hawai'i was just sixteen at the end of April. At the hospital, politics were put aside, teamwork prevailed, and the house Queen Emma built stood proud, guarding the town. ଔ

Chapter Seven

THE AMERICAN DESCENT

MAY 31, 2020

643 HAWAIʻI	
1,716,078 UNITED STATES	5,934,195 WORLD

COVID-19 cases (data sources: World Health Organization and Hawaii Department of Health)

As the haze of novelty lifted in April and May, it became apparent that Hawaiʻi was in better shape than most states on the Mainland. The epidemic had peaked small and left quickly. The restrictions on transpacific flight, combined with the lockdown orders, were just in time to have their intended effect. Bruce Soll, a mentor and colleague in pulmonary medicine, posited that the weather (in particular the temperature and relative humidity) could make community transmission in Hawaiʻi more difficult. This fit with another theory gaining traction, that vitamin D levels (higher in the tropics) protected against the infection. It was a fact that the state had many visitors in February, and yet a relatively small epidemic in March and April.

As the year progressed, unexpectedly mild epidemics would occur in a few other regions, mostly near the equator. Sub-Saharan Africa, with its dense urban centers and poor infrastructure, was an area of early concern for disease modelers. But ultimately the mortality event in Africa was small, with the notable exception of South Africa. Likewise, India initially had a small mortality event compared to its population size. Antibody studies suggested the pandemic reached these places and spread widely through urban populations, but it didn't translate into full hospitals or large numbers of deaths. And yet in some warm countries, like Mexico and Brazil, it did. As Siddhartha Mukherjee has pointed out, this remains one of the unsolved mysteries of the pandemic.

I was interested in these ideas, and in any factor that could improve success against the virus, but I didn't think it wise to trust Hawai'i's safety in weather or latitude. In April, a COVID epidemic gripped Guayaquil, Ecuador, a city located on the equator, and it mercilessly killed thousands of residents. The bodies piled up so fast in that town that they couldn't bury them, or count cases, and the *New York Times* posted pictures of corpses left on the street with cardboard covering them. The world was soon to see further examples of geographic variation in attack rates that did not correlate in any clean or direct way with latitude. Ultimately Miami, Florida, had as high a mortality rate as Philadelphia, Pennsylvania. Anchorage, Alaska, would do almost as well as Honolulu.

There likely is a benefit to warm climate, and the vitamin D literature is intriguing (deficiency in the vitamin is correlated with a worse clinical course for a number of infections), but indoor crowding is the most relevant factor for disease transmission of SARS-CoV-2. Honolulu has one of the highest rates in the country of crowded and multigenerational homes. It's also the case that many Hawai'i residents, despite living in the tropics, do not have high vitamin D levels. I thought the risk of a severe epidemic was present, especially in the more urban parts of Honolulu.

As the pandemic wore on, I frequently heard people assert that this or that factor was most important in controlling spread. Some advised everyone to take vitamin D supplements. Others made it a point to emphasize mask wearing. Identify the key factor, the thinking went, and crush the epidemic. There was reasonableness to these views, as each identified item had a basis in the medical literature and could, applied appropriately, contribute to a successful strategy. But the notion that experts could reduce risk to any one thing struck me as naïve. Mark

Crislip, who publishes an excellent podcast reviewing the infectious diseases literature, has long observed that infections are multifactorial in their etiology. In the struggle against SARS-CoV-2, this was certainly the case, and the ability to react to events with a nimble and targeted public health system, and to address vulnerabilities in real time, was more important than modifying any single factor.

It's also true that chance is a part of viral transmission. Just as it's inevitable that a respiratory virus will spread through a nonimmune population given enough time, it's equally true that the virus is under no obligation to arrive when and where you expect it. It's not making a reservation. It doesn't read disease models or watch the weather channel, and it doesn't care about expert opinion, which is often wrong for new diseases. In the case of Hawai'i, it's likely that infected tourists missed locals in the majority of their social interactions. As I saw on the wards, traveling locals who were infected passed the disease to their relatives, and so Hawai'i saw a different epidemic than I was expecting. Fortunately for the state, it was a smaller one.

The shutdowns in April had wide public support, and almost everyone I knew wanted to help. After years of living in sequestered media bubbles and avoiding each other, the outpouring of community effort to beat back the virus was refreshing. It proved to me that people were, despite the ugly fragmentation of American society, craving a sense of shared identity. And they wanted leadership.

But that's not what they got. The national response to COVID was a disaster. There was no organized approach to testing, and there was no attempt to coordinate a public health response across state boundaries. Testing was also not linked in any coherent way to contact tracing or quarantine. The result was that the US, which eventually generated massive testing numbers, never had an integrated or effective response.

More importantly, the organizational failures reflected political attitudes. The president made it clear from early on that he wanted the virus to go away as a policy issue. Initially, he was more concerned with the stock market. Later, as his re-election prospects dimmed, it was the job market. He vacillated wildly between testing more and testing less. Some moments he was a "war president," but during others he spread self-pitying theories that the subject was a plot to make him unpopular. Morally speaking, he was a small man, and he never accepted the premise that to lead the country he had to do competent things to control the disease.

The president was just one face of the political right. The disease was the ultimate refutation of the small government philosophy, because it demanded a massive investment in services like public health, which conservatives opposed for ideological reasons. Libertarians like Senator Rand Paul seemed frustrated that the virus hadn't read Ayn Rand, and they made a habit of demanding irrational sacrifices of their voters. Paul, an eye doctor who skipped his boards, jumped the queue to get himself tested in March. He then failed to self-isolate while awaiting his (positive) result. This experience humbled him not a bit, and he made a habit of pontificating to Anthony Fauci on disease control measures. Like many on the libertarian right, he didn't seem aware that it was his politics, not the science of epidemiology, that was on trial before the public, or that he was flailing badly. There was no inkling of self-awareness, no ability to self-correct. He was, as I observed to friends, "a perfect hot air balloon."

Many on the conservative right avoided Paul's contempt for Fauci, but simply could not make the mental adjustment necessary to spend billions (or even trillions) of dollars coordinating a federal response. The virus, unconcerned with politics, simply exploited the holes.

Despite the failure of Republicans to meet the moment, I thought it was dishonest to focus on Trump, who was floundering, and ignore the deficiencies of liberal states and institutions. New York was not the only debacle. California liberals faired just as poorly. After enacting a series of business-crushing restrictions, Governor Gavin Newsom visited an expensive restaurant—without wearing a mask—and dined with a lobbyist. San Francisco mayor London Breed attended a party at the same restaurant. Even House Speaker Nancy Pelosi got her hair done indoors at a salon, when San Francisco salons were supposed to be closed to indoor business. And while they managed to hurt small business and antagonize their citizens, California Democrats ultimately didn't put a dent in viral transmission.

The failures in California were not only symbolic ones. Although they locked down early in the spring and had great success crushing their initial wave, the state's reopening suffered from inconsistencies that angered local residents. This included opening malls while schools remained shuttered, a problem that was later to hurt public support for liberal governments in many states, including Hawaiʻi. California also suffered a scandal in which their unemployment office paid billions of dollars in fraudulent benefits, while millions of Californians couldn't access the system. In this context of failing to deliver services like education and unemployment support, the luxuries taken by California's political class reinforced the perception that leaders were self-interested and incompetent.

California would end up with large surges of cases in both the summer and winter. They had the most deaths in the country, with hospitals in Los Angeles severely taxed even months after being resupplied with critical equipment. If indifference doomed Trump, it was hypocrisy and ineptitude that doomed many Democrats.

Within the federal government, the CDC stumbled from one failure to the next. They allowed political pressure from the White House to water down their guidelines for reopening the economy, including schools. Later they changed their recommendations on testing close contacts to exclude asymptomatic relatives, a stance that made no sense if the goal was to control an infection with a large number of asymptomatic carriers. Their director, Robert Redfield, was a lamb occupying the position of a lion. At crucial moments, he simply disappeared, allowing the president's political appointees to overshadow him. For the CDC, the early testing disaster was a bad blow, but the series of damaging and self-contradicting recommendations eventually caused the public, as well as many doctors, to tune them out altogether.

An early but important example of the confused messaging from the federal government pertained to mask use. In February and March, authorities recommended against the public purchasing masks. This was in contrast to Asian countries, which masked up quickly when the threat from the virus became clear. There were two distinct issues at play. One was confusion over the utility of masks for preventing transmission. The other was a concern over the supply of masks. But these points became muddled, and as the supply of masks improved, the recommendation shifted in April. Suddenly everyone needed a mask, and even a home-made cloth mask was better than nothing.

Zeynep Tufecki, an associate professor at UNC-Chapel Hill whose work specializes in digital technology and misinformation, wrote an op-ed column in the *New York Times* in mid-March that impacted the rule change. Alarmed by the poor state of public health communication, she wrote that "of course masks work—maybe not perfectly and not all to the same degree, but they provide some protection." Having made a close study of the successful response in Asia, she had a better grasp of the situation than many epidemiologists. But weeks of false reassurance to the public that they don't need masks had already done damage to the credibility of the experts.

There's a lesson to be learned here about the value of honest and humble communication during an emergency. Any concerns about supply should have been communicated clearly, not used as the basis for erroneous recommendations. If there was uncertainty about the value of masks, that too should have been part of the communication. But health authorities in Asia had no such uncertainty, and they were right. My own impression was that the public was eager to contribute, and the vast majority would have shared rather than hoarded masks if approached in an honest way. Instead, the government condescended to them.

It was the shocking failure of liberal government, and institutions long associated with the liberal project, that made a profound impression on me. Trump benefited from the low expectations everyone had of him. But for the CDC and other federal institutions to nosedive into irrelevance at the moment when their leadership was most critical was unforgivable. It played into the narrative that government couldn't be trusted, a long-standing assertion of the conservative right—and a self-fulfilling prophecy that made the pandemic worse than it had to be.

One frustrating example of pandemic politics took the form of arguments over the fatality rate of the infection. In my initial post warning of the pandemic, I made a caveat, which was that if the infection proved to be far less fatal than had been reported, that would be a legitimate cause to lower my concern. When I said this, on February 29,

I was just trying to keep myself honest. Having raised the alarm in such a public way, I thought I owed readers an explanation of my thinking, as well as a comment on what would change it.

This presaged a contentious argument over the deadliness of the infection that would consume months of attention from some of America's most prominent scientists. In the end, it was a debate that created more smoke than light, and it accomplished nothing useful.

One source of smoke was confusion over the difference between case fatality rate (CFR) and infection fatality rate (IFR). The CFR simply divided COVID deaths by confirmed COVID cases in a given area. When discussing the severity of an epidemic, it's the CFR that's often used. The IFR measures deaths divided by total cases of disease (including those not picked up through diagnostic testing). This is a much trickier number to pin down. However, with COVID it soon became apparent that a majority of cases were either asymptomatic or mildly symptomatic, and many of these people couldn't access molecular testing. If they developed immunity to the disease, but were undiagnosed, that was certainly relevant in understanding the severity of the epidemic. This is why attempts to clarify the IFR were reasonable.

Unfortunately, the legitimate scientific discussion in this realm quickly became overshadowed by politics. A paper from Santa Clara, California, which used antibody tests to estimate how many people were truly infected in the county, suggested a much more widespread (and mild) epidemic. The methods of this study quickly came under question for technical reasons, but that didn't stop the political right from making it a major news item. Soon afterwards it became impossible to have sane conversations about the IFR, as people on either side of the political divide cherry-picked studies that showed their preferred outcome.

The truth is that using antibody tests to precisely pin down the infection fatality rate always involved a fudge factor, due to the performance characteristics of those tests and how the sampling was conducted. But I thought this conversation had become asinine. We knew only a minority of New Yorkers had become infected in March and April, likely no more than 25 percent. With tens of thousands of deaths in New York, and the hospital system overwhelmed, I didn't need an IFR calculation to tell me the epidemic was severe.

I suspect there will still be arguments over IFR years after the epidemic ends. Given the geographic and temporal variability of the illness, it may ultimately make most sense to speak of IFRs (plural), correlating with different waves of illness in different communities. My own best estimate, from reading analyses of the better-conducted studies, is that it ranges from 0.2 to 0.8 percent. That means SARS-CoV-2 is an order of magnitude worse than influenza, but not nearly as bad as its cousin coronaviruses, SARS-CoV-1 or MERS. But even that number reflects a tremendous amount of age stratification. The disease is more deadly in the elderly than the young. It can also rocket upwards in situations where healthcare capacity is overwhelmed, as was seen in Italy and New York.

These subtleties weren't of much interest to people who were determined, for ideological reasons, to promote whatever talking point was most convenient.

In early summer, the virus entered an ugly plateau of about twenty thousand cases per day nationally, far too many to be safe or in the clear, and that's when the economic fallout began to bite. Tens of millions of people were out of work. This was a shock that made the economic crisis of 2008 paltry in comparison. Without a robust safety net, and with no prospect of the government controlling the disease, desperation began to grow. It was a racist police killing that proved to be the spark. The murder of George Floyd by a Minnesota police officer, captured on video, led to massive national street protests. For thousands of people, this was their first social interaction in months. The majority of protesters were peaceful, but a few engaged in vandalism. This prompted counter-protests and police tactics that often resulted in violence. In Seattle, a protest zone "liberated" a commercial portion of that city. After a string of violent incidents, capped by two murders, the police moved in to break up the anarchy. The president took advantage of the chaos to portray himself as the voice of law and order. If he couldn't beat the virus, he could at least beat the protesters.

The argument that soon erupted in academic circles was another signpost indicating the breakdown of sane conversation. In June, a letter endorsing the protests was signed by over a thousand physicians, public health officials, and epidemiologists. This created some stir, as the public health talking point for months had been that people should avoid gathering. In a subsequent piece published by *The Atlantic*, Julia Marcus and Gregg Gonsalves (epidemiologists from Harvard and Yale, respectively) explained their stance. They argued that "systemic racism" was as much a public health concern as the pandemic. The pandemic had just killed a hundred thousand people in three months. It would soon kill half a million. To people who asked if endorsing large gatherings sent a mixed message, they dismissed the concerns as "a call to color blindness."

I felt sympathy for the protesters, the vast majority of whom were in pain over an abuse of authority they recognized all too well. Most protesters wore masks and took precautions not to transmit the disease. The Black congressional leadership also behaved soberly, focusing on police reforms that would help their community. But I felt differently about my colleagues in academia. There I saw hypocrisy masquerading as virtue. Heavy on politics and light on consistency, the endorsement of gatherings was a pose that was poison for creating any communal approach to the pandemic. The result was that it further diminished the authority of the experts, whom the conservative half of the country viewed as hostile. As those Americans increasingly turned away from science, they encountered people who were unencumbered by the facts of the disease, and they acted on the bad ideas they consumed. That, too, was a public health outcome.

It was during this dreary descent into faction and conformity, pursued by both extremes of the political spectrum, that the philosopher and neuroscientist Sam Harris made what I thought was a useful contribution to the conversation:

> I'll tell you the fear of the other that does seem warranted, everywhere, right now. It's the other who has rendered him or herself incapable of dialogue. It's the other who will not listen to reason, who has no interest in facts, who can't join a conversation that converges on the truth, because he knows in advance what the truth must be. We should fear the other who thinks dogmatism and cognitive bias aren't something to be corrected for, because they're the very foundations of his epistemology. We should fear the other who can't distinguish activism from journalism or politics from science. Or worse, can make these distinctions, but

refuses to. And we're all capable of becoming this person. If only for minutes or hours at a time. And this is a bug in our operating system, not a feature. We have to continually correct for it.

In the wake of this fragmentation, increasingly surreal conspiracy theories spread about the disease and about physicians. Many conspiracies targeted Anthony Fauci, who had for decades led the National Institute of Allergy and Infectious Diseases. Fauci was, before the pandemic, a fixture at the Infectious Diseases Society of America (IDSA) meetings. I found him an engaging speaker, and I remember in particular a talk in San Diego in 2017 when he described the acceleration in vaccine development time. This proved a critical factor in the spring of 2020, and he was obviously the right man to have on hand.

Fauci was not perfect, and in February he made a few comments that appeared to downplay the risk of the virus. He was also part of the hasty U-turn on mask wearing. But he adjusted as his own grasp of the data improved and the seriousness of the situation became apparent. He had a number of sober interactions with the press, and he filled the information void left by the CDC during the early days of the pandemic. His demeanor was always calm, and when politics happened around him, as it often did, he became amused rather than angry. This was exactly the right tone to strike. In one *Saturday Night Live* sketch, Brad Pitt portrayed the famous doctor, who opened fan mail that included lingerie from elderly women. But this popularity made him a threat to Trump, and the conspiracy theorists alleged that he exaggerated the pandemic to boost his own government agency. He soon became unwelcome in the White House, where an overtly politicized response had become policy, and where idolization of Trump began to take on a cult-like quality.

My own favorite conspiracy was that doctors (working in silent but perfect coordination) overcounted cases, listing all patients as COVID cases, in order to increase medical reimbursements. My practice had lost about 30 percent of its revenue since the pandemic began, due to the shutdown of elective medical care, and I wondered aloud to my colleagues how I could access this treasure trove of fraudulent billing.

A common stupidity of this time was, "he died with COVID, but not of COVID." Basic statistics were no longer trusted, and no amount of effort to redirect people with facts could restore trust. The denial that allowed people to board airplanes without masks allowed them to explain away deaths, in some cases in their own family, as having nothing to do with the new disease. The actuarial data showed the truth, which was that the United States was experiencing a severe mortality event, with hundreds of thousands of "excess deaths" over the 2019 total, correlating closely with the pandemic death count.

But increasingly, America resembled a Soviet-like state, where the truth was processed for media consumption rather than reported plainly to help people understand events. Constant spin, denial, demagogic rhetoric, and conspiracy thinking—mediated through the internet and cable news—became the preferred form of social interaction for tens of millions of people, who of course lacked access to real social interaction.

The most chilling thing about the pandemic was the way it layered so neatly onto America's societal dysfunction. A health crisis became an economic crisis, which became a race crisis, which became a political crisis. And then the long-smoldering distrust between Americans ignited and became open hostility. Old problems, unsolved, transfigured into ghastly new ones. I had a newfound understanding of the ancient Athenians, who were toppled by a plague at the height of their power. I rediscovered the essays of Marcus Aurelius, who patrolled the crumbling frontier of the Roman Empire during the Antonine Plague, which killed millions and ended the epoch of Roman greatness. I read a history of the bubonic plague, which killed almost half of Europe in the fourteenth century and marked the terminus of the Middle Ages. In each case, infection worked as an accelerant, aggravating social conflict and disrupting institutions that had become inflexible and corrupt.

Civilization is fragile, and history is a ravine littered with the corpses of states sent careening over the edge by epidemic disease. Infection acts not just on human bodies, but on human ignorance.

Chapter Eight

HAWAI'I VICTORIOUS

In May, Hawai'i enjoyed a strange interlude, where the disease retreated from the Islands but the Mainland slipped further into chaos. The juxtaposition of life here and there unsettled me. In Hawai'i, there were days with no cases and many days with only one or two. The government began lifting restrictions, and people resumed daily life. I remember the first time I had a friend over. Layla and I greeted her in the backyard and had a drink at a distance of about ten feet. Masks were now standard, and we were all adjusting to their use in daily life.

On the Mainland, millions of people rejected mask use, subscribing to conspiracy theories and suspect interpretations of the Constitution. It became yet another culture war issue for the far right, where the lack of mask wearing signaled one's commitment to personal freedom. After watching the ICU begin to fill up, I saw gestures such as these as ignorant. Fortunately, there were few people in Hawai'i who rejected respiratory hygiene in order to express their political identity. But the mere fact that this happened—and the scale at which it occurred in the rest of the country—was evidence of the further unmooring from reality of millions of Americans.

I was further alarmed by the condition of the Department of Health. They had failed to support testing early on O'ahu and had only been saved by the efforts of private labs. Chris Whelen at Diagnostic Lab Services (DLS) provided most of the testing for the Queen's system. Scott Miscovich, a doctor who ran a number of primary care clinics in the community, arranged drive-in testing on the Korean model. He sent his swabs to Clinical Labs of Hawaii (CLH), another private lab, and this effort tested thousands more people. Without these private efforts, I am convinced Hawai'i would have been hearing "the risk is low" as the ICUs filled up.

The DOH dysfunction ran deeper than testing problems. In talking to patients admitted during April, it became clear that interactions with the DOH contact tracing staff were superficial, and there was no regular use of hotel rooms for isolation and quarantine. The state wasn't testing. It wasn't contact tracing. And it wasn't performing isolation or quarantine. So what was it doing? The issue of quarantine had been the cause of my fallout with HI-EMA. It was easy with cases dropping due to the lockdown to pretend that everything was well. But the combination of failed public health measures was a guillotine perched above the state's neck.

I had daily conversations with my hui, who saw the problems plainly. David Derauf was my principal ally, but with increasing regularity we spoke with Jerry Murphy, Tim Brown, and Chad Meyer. Tim brought with him DeWolfe Miller, the state's preeminent epidemiologist and an emeritus professor at the University of Hawai'i Mānoa. He also partnered with Sumner La Croix, a retired professor of economics and fellow at the UH Economic Research Organization (UHERO). The seven of us covered a broad range of clinical and academic expertise, and we had contacts in every part of the healthcare sector, government, media, and business communities. I began thinking of us as an informal think tank, a kind of shadow cabinet for Governor Ige's public health bureaucracy.

It was David who suggested we speak with Sarah Park. Park was the state epidemiologist, and alongside Bruce Anderson, she was the principal director of the Health Department. Our disagreement with the DOH was so profound that I thought an effort to clear the air worthwhile. I had met Park once previously while establishing the antimicrobial stewardship program at Queen's. I knew she was bright. I thought there must be some misunderstanding, or she must know something important that I was missing. Maybe she was under great strain and needed professional support. I wanted us to drop the acrimony and help her.

It was in that spirit I entered the conversation. David invited me and Jerry, and we set a time for a call. But right from the start it went off the rails. Park expressed frustration at the expectation that she test more widely, insisting that this wasn't based on the science. She was angry with Scott Miscovich, who had criticized her department. Jerry pushed back in his mild way, pointing out that Miscovich was popular because he had stepped into a void and provided a necessary service. But this made little impression. Her animosity towards broader testing was evident, and her interpretation of the science was fixed. I didn't say much. It was clear to me that our support was welcome, but not our collaboration. The call ended politely, and we briefly discussed speaking again. But I was troubled at how she had staked out such an isolated position.

In retrospect, this moment was a failure in the state's disease control effort, not technically, but culturally. Looking around at my own circle, I saw a group of doctors criticizing the state response, although at that time mostly we criticized it in private. Here on the state side was a fellow infectious diseases doctor. She was obviously talented, with a tremendous knowledge base, and she was struggling against a monstrous challenge. My desire was to help her. I would have been pleased if she joined our group's regular conversations, or if we could bring resources to lighten her load. Working together we could have swept all before us. But I encountered a wall, and my colleagues had a similar impression. From that time forward, until the DOH leadership changed in September, our relations were adversarial.

During the quarantine troubles in April, David and I began speaking with representatives of Mayor Kirk Caldwell. Josh Stanbro was the city sustainability officer, and Hiro Toiya ran emergency response. These were key figures in the city government, and they helped obtain hotel rooms for some COVID patients. Soon they invited us to join a new medical advisory group assisting the city with its COVID response.

The mayor's medical advisory group first met on April 16. This was my first impression of Kirk Caldwell. He attended the entire meeting, and he continued to chair weekly or biweekly meetings for the duration of his term. His availability to clinical physicians distinguished him from the state leadership. Not only that, but he showed interest in the medical and scientific issues underlying the pandemic response. He often read articles and came with pointed questions. It was clear that he was trying to stake out his own ground on pandemic response, and he wanted a solid footing in the science.

His questions were fresh air, and his demeanor furthered this impression. He could be funny, at times self-deprecating, and this created an easy forum for us to discuss matters frankly. He also showed an interest in each person offering him their time. He wanted to know about my school experiences and my house on the Big Island. I found myself liking him immediately, and though I was aware that this was a politician's art, I let myself enjoy his new group.

David and I were regulars on the mayor's calls, and this was how I met Libby Char. Libby is an ER doctor who worked at the city and helped coordinate the fire department's medical response. She eschewed the spotlight and was quiet during the first few meetings. But she perceived quickly the deficiencies of the state's public health response. At times, she would say out loud what many people were thinking. The conversation would pause, briefly, and then go in a new and more honest direction. In those moments, which she never drew attention to, she would lead the group.

Another member was Al Katz, a public health expert at UH Mānoa, who also ran the venereal diseases clinic at Diamond Head. He was one of many doctors who trained me during residency, the only person I ever swabbed a penis with. That's a bond unique to the medical arts. He had the right sense of humor for his job and decades of experience in disease response. I was glad to see him, and in the new crisis I drew reassurance from reconnecting with a mentor.

The DOH liaison to the mayor's team was Liz MacNeill, who ran their TB control branch. I knew her from clinical work at Queen's. I thought her an excellent TB doctor. I viewed her inclusion as a fortuitous choice, especially after the conversation with Sarah Park. But when I reached out to her by text to discuss the new group, and the problems I saw arising, she let the topic drop. I wondered if I already had a reputation. This left me no choice but to ask in public about issues I intended to discuss in private.

My attempts to find a sympathetic ear at the DOH were, at that point, unsuccessful. MacNeill was open-minded and could admit to problems at the Health Department, but she was not their chief. Their leadership culture prevented any real reckoning, even with the mayor present. MacNeill was often caught in the middle, working long hours and relaying information she didn't necessarily agree with, a position that was unfair to her and untenable. She later returned to the TB branch, where she did excellent work. I would have done the same in her place.

I'll give two examples of the rising tension between city and state.

The mayor complained that he wasn't receiving timely and detailed information on where cases were occurring. The Health Department responded that they could not share detailed information with the city because the city people would "leak" the information. This concern for preventing leaks, rather than communicating clearly with the public, epitomized the DOH administration's approach.

Later, when the second wave was upon us, I expressed dismay that so many hotel rooms were empty while cases piled up in multigenerational apartments. The DOH had still not adjusted their approach to quarantine. They replied that they weren't giving "vacation rooms" to people who could stay home. I found this appalling. Honolulu's Pacific Islander community, many working-class and poor, were infecting each other in crowded housing. But officials working for the state dismissed them as angling for free benefits. The racial overtone was ugly, and David and I kept beating the quarantine drum. We wanted not just access to hotel rooms for these patients, but also access to financial support and wraparound services, so that they could stay home from work while sick.

A dynamic emerged during these meetings in which the jurisdiction of the city, represented by Caldwell, chafed against that of the state. Over time I became one of the more vocal proponents of city action. I was agnostic about the jurisdictional question. I would have been happy to see the state take on its natural role. They were simply refusing to do so. When you are in a life-and-death struggle, you pull any useful lever, and I thought the city owed the state no apology for intruding on their turf. The only thing that mattered to me was that we kick the virus, and keep kicking it. The city lawyers often attended these meetings, and I would have given them plenty of work defending the mayor's initiatives in court. As the state's obstruction went on, the mayor went well beyond simply pushing the DOH for answers. He stood up testing, he invested in quarantine rooms for sick patients, and he eventually hired his own contact tracers. There was even brief talk of setting up a city health department so that Honolulu could take its fate into its own hands. No doubt that would have raised constitutional questions about who in Hawaiʻi is responsible for public health. But courtroom drama proved to be unnecessary. In the end, city and state healed their rift, which was the best outcome.

Despite these problems, the early summer was a victory party for Hawaiʻi. People poured outside after weeks of lockdown. Barbecues and beach gatherings resumed in earnest. The dreadful news from the Mainland couldn't penetrate the fun, and my stomach sank as I began to see large groups gather under beach tents, in the parks, and around youth baseball games. The fun outside wasn't too dangerous, but it reflected a false confidence, and it correlated with increasingly large gatherings inside.

People in Hawaiʻi had cooperated with the shutdown and shown genuine patriotism. But as spring turned to summer, pandemic fatigue became a real phenomenon. Conspiracy theories common on the Mainland gained traction locally, and there was a new sense of resentment any time an authority discussed restricting an activity. I remember a particular interaction that was notable for its insanity. A young woman, staff at the hospital, asked me if I had watched a YouTube video asserting the pandemic was exaggerated. I responded that I didn't need YouTube to help me with that, because I could walk up a flight of stairs and see the patients. I invited her to see for herself. Her eyes bulged, and she shook her head incredulously. I clearly didn't get it. As she shuffled off, she advised me to educate myself properly online.

During this interlude, the mayor came under tremendous pressure from businesses to reopen everything, including high-transmission venues like bars. The religious community was vocal and insisted on indoor, in-person gatherings. The medical advisory group, almost without exception, thought these activities should not happen. But I, too, was sensitive to the suffering of my neighbors, and no one liked the idea of imposing restrictions on small congregations and businesses. The advisory group suggested a gradual reopening, with low-risk venues before high risk. I thought backtracking was nothing to be ashamed of if the situation dictated it. This was a death match, and public health measures were the mayor's only weapons. He needed the flexibility to move wherever the struggle took him. But that kind of nuance was absent from the broader conversation. People expected unreasonable consistency in response to a virus whose biology scientists were still learning.

With the numbers low in May, and testing capacity briefly in excess, I wished for an aggressive surveillance program to test asymptomatic people in high-risk areas. In particular I wanted to test all healthcare workers, first responders, nursing home residents, prisoners, homeless people in shelters, and people in public housing. The last group was of particular concern given the dense congregate living in Kalihi and Pālolo, and the comorbid medical illnesses in that population. David had flagged this in our first conversation.

In pushing this approach, I was cognizant of the example of Singapore. The island city had started the year a paragon of success for its SARS-CoV-2 containment effort. One of the first countries impacted as the disease spread outside China, Singapore had one of the best records for containment. The strategy relied on test-trace-isolate techniques, combined with a high level of mutual cooperation between the government and citizens. For the first few months of the pandemic, Singapore managed to avoid a lockdown and keep its economy, including schools, open.

But there was a population of workers in Singapore that few officials there wished to acknowledge. The city hosted hundreds of thousands of "guest workers," migrants from poorer countries in Asia, who worked jobs in construction and manufacturing. These workers had no minimum wage, and they lived in dormitories that housed multiple people per room. Like Dorian Gray's portrait rotting in the closet, there was an ugly reality concealed by Singapore's wealth.

When the virus reached these dormitories, Singapore experienced over a thousand cases per day, and its reputation for disease control was shattered. The news also drew attention to the plight of its often-ignored workforce, much of which was moved into hastily constructed "community care beds" in public buildings. The outbreak was concentrated amongst the foreign workers, but the disease forced the entire island to enter lockdown.

Singapore's experience was repeated throughout the world wherever there were neglected populations in dense, congregate living. In the United States, this meant prisons, where it proved impossible to keep the virus at bay. I wished to apply these lessons to Honolulu, in the hope of preventing a Singapore-style meltdown amongst the poorest residents.

The city had difficulty targeting testing to the areas where it would have been most helpful. The lack of an effective strategy to screen asymptomatic, high-risk people is attributable to a few causes. The Health Department was hostile to the concept. Engagement with the highest-risk communities required time and relationships built over weeks to months, as well as support services for patients. Testing resources were only briefly in excess, with cases on the Mainland straining supply chains. Finally, there was the unwillingness of private insurance to reimburse the cost of screening tests.

The virus didn't care about this dysfunction. It simply continued to spread, though at a reduced level, and slip through the cracks left open for it. It would soon make its way into both public housing and prisons. But in the early summer, there were few people worrying about the next round. Hawaiʻi indulged a mood of self-satisfaction, and the state lost a window of opportunity, one that disappeared all too quickly, to eradicate the virus from the Islands. ☙

Chapter Nine

PROTECTING THESE ISLANDS

JUNE 30, 2020

907
HAWAIʻI

2,537,636	**10,185,633**
UNITED STATES	WORLD

COVID-19 cases (data sources: World Health Organization and Hawaii Department of Health)

My frustration in failing to ramp up testing for high-risk, asymptomatic people represented a small corner of a larger, national debate about testing. By early spring, with hospitals in New York full, it was clear that testing for symptomatic disease was a critical task. Hawaiʻi's use of private labs to do that testing, before disease became deeply entrenched, enabled the state to define and contain the first wave of infection. Testing close contacts of symptomatic cases, regardless of their symptoms, was also becoming standard practice in most of the world. Given the growing literature on asymptomatic infection, and documented transmission of virus from asymptomatic patients to their contacts, any well-coordinated effort to contain COVID-19 needed to include testing close contacts of identified patients. Here the Hawaii Department of Health opposed testing, insisting that as long as contacts quarantined at home, they didn't need to test them.

I disagreed with that. But I also wanted something more radical. I wanted large-scale testing of asymptomatic people regardless of whether they were in contact with a known case. I wanted to see access to testing for anyone in a high-risk setting (e.g. healthcare, jail, public housing, etc.). The purpose of such a program would be to make those high-risk settings safer. Furthermore, I thought the scale of testing should be so vast that the involvement of doctors would be unnecessary.

I was committing a heresy. The traditional medical model of testing is that a physician orders a test on an individual patient based on signs and symptoms, and that doctor is then responsible for interpreting and acting on the result. But jettisoning that paradigm was not an act of sloppiness. I drew the idea from some of the brightest academics in the country, who were calling for a new approach. In particular I was influenced by the work of Harvard's Michael Mina and Fred Hutchinson's Trevor Bedford.

Their idea was to expand testing on such a scale that it could be used regularly by a significant portion of the population in order to open (and keep open) critical industries. Rather than requiring a doctor visit, followed by a few hundred dollars of lab work, the idea was to make testing so available and so cheap that it could be done repeatedly. This would require a massive upscaling of testing resources. Bedford referred to it as "the Apollo program of our times." But crucially, it would require a change in the way doctors think about testing.

Under ordinary circumstances, parsimony is a virtue. Tests are expensive, and I should have a good reason for ordering one. If it's unlikely to change management, or if my pretest suspicion is low, I should avoid ordering the test. A doctor who orders a bunch of tests that come back normal receives a kind of academic scolding, like a child who has gluttoned himself on leftover birthday cake. Over-testing is also a common criticism of the defensive medical model, and it's viewed as a contributor to cost overruns in American medicine.

This was the attitude that Mina and Bedford wanted to retire. In the new paradigm, the purpose of testing had nothing to do with an individual patient–doctor encounter. The doctor was almost completely irrelevant (a fact that in itself explained a lot of the hostility to the concept). Rather, the goal was to provide people participating in critical activities (e.g. school, trancontinental travel, or critical infrastructure work) access to a cheap test, with reasonable sensitivity, that could be repeated at multiple time points. In other words, the goal was to create security at a population level, not an individual level, so that key activities could remain open.

As with any imperfect strategy for fighting the pandemic, this one had its warts. It would take time to scale up testing to a point where it could be used on asymptomatic people in this way. Handling the enormous amount of information generated would create its own problems. Who would follow up on a positive test result if the test was not ordered by a doctor? If testing would be used on such an enormous scale, inevitably there would be more false positives than true positives. Someone would have to sort that out as well. Most importantly, the existing tests had been designed for use in symptomatic disease, so their performance characteristics for asymptomatic screening were largely unknown.

I thought all these problems were solvable, and the various "bubbles" based on serial testing that industry later created around sports leagues, Hollywood sets, and other businesses showed their practicality. I admired Mina and Bedford for promoting an innovative approach. The country needed creative solutions, ones with the potential to disrupt the forward progress of the pandemic, and it was also important for morale to change the terms of the competition with the virus. The alternative, which involved shutting down entire segments of the economy for months on end, struck me as too bleak and provided an excellent incentive to try.

There was at least one entrepreneur in Hawai'i who shared my view of the situation. Patrick Sullivan, the CEO of Oceanit, had long dreamed of building a tech industry in Hawai'i. In his book, *Intellectual Anarchy: The Art of Disruptive Innovation*, written just before the pandemic, he argues against the notion that geography must determine economic possibilities. He asserts that new technology, including 3D printing, allows manufacturing to happen almost anywhere. The key ingredient is human capital, as well as a cultural willingness to take risks. Sullivan wrote a chapter analyzing the problem with "expert thinking." He took care to point out the valuable contributions of experts. They could often tell him how best to do a thing and save him time and money doing it. But the pitfall with experts often comes with their assessment of what cannot be done, which he tends to distrust. No innovation is possible unless science goes beyond the bounds of known practice, and so it's foolish to allow experts to confine a conversation to the tasks they have already mastered.

Sullivan's assessment matched comments I had heard from other successful entrepreneurs, including Elon Musk, who famously quipped that he fires experts who don't try to innovate beyond their base of knowledge. The fact that this approach fails more often than it succeeds is not a flaw but an expected cost of operating business in a way that is "disruptive" of existing technical and economic structures.

Oceanit is an engineering firm, working on everything from diving helmets to artificial intelligence. They have numerous contracts on the Mainland and around the world and have been a regular participant in Defense Department competitions for technological innovation. Disruption is a deliberate part of their business strategy. Their involvement in biotech arose out of artificial intelligence software they developed for cancer research to help decrypt gene sequencing data. When the pandemic hit, the Oceanit team shifted their focus to the virus.

Sullivan's first effort was a simple one. Partnering with colleagues in Korea, he tried to get five hundred thousand test kits for the state. As these were from Korea, they lacked FDA authorization, but they were approved by the WHO. He even arranged funding for the kits. He was surprised to find that the state wasn't interested in acquiring them.

It's worth taking a moment to pause at the mentality that would turn down hundreds of thousands of free test kits at a time when testing resources were severely limited. Here was an opportunity for Hawaiʻi to implement an early version of the Mina strategy, or at least to insure itself against a future disruption in the testing supply chain. But it would have required some awkward conversations with the FDA, and likely a research protocol to validate the tests and establish a legal framework for their use. Most importantly, it would have required a desire to actually find the disease. That effectively killed it.

Sullivan then shifted gears, and he began the work of producing his own test kit. Familiar with the ideas of Mina, Oceanit opted for a lateral flow assay (LFA), instead of a nucleic acid amplification test (NAAT). Unlike NAATs, which include the polymerase chain reaction (PCR) tests most commonly in use, a lateral flow assay doesn't require sophisticated lab equipment. There's no need to amplify viral RNA, or to control temperature through thermal cycling. Instead, the person being tested provides a saliva sample, and it simply detects the presence of viral antigen. A bar on a piece of paper changes color to indicate the antigen is present. It functions like a home pregnancy test.

The beauty of antigen tests is they are cheap, ranging from around five to twenty-five dollars per test, and can be produced at massive scale. This solves one of the critical problems identified in screening asymptomatic people. Michael Mina, in particular, has been a major advocate of their adoption to widescale use. Antigen tests may actually be better than the more sensitive NAATs for screening large populations, because they only turn positive at higher levels of viral shedding, which correspond with contagiousness. The more sensitive NAATs, on the other hand, would inappropriately stay positive long after a patient has recovered.

Sullivan's LFA has one additional advantage, in my eyes, which is that the antigen tested is the virus nucleocapsid protein. This means that the test should work well against virus that has mutations in the spike protein. As a means of opening up a critical industry, like air travel, cheap and repeatable tests like the Oceanit LFA could reassure the state that it's not importing mutant strains of SARS-CoV-2.

But here, too, Sullivan hit a wall, at least temporarily. To produce the test locally, he needed a clean room with low humidity, and Oceanit sought a contract from the state. The governor, likely influenced by the advice of his health department, backed out of any final decision. Oceanit is now looking to complete FDA approval for their test, and unless there's new interest from Hawai'i, they will manufacture it elsewhere. That's five hundred to a thousand biotechnology and construction jobs that will go to another state.

The frustrations of the Oceanit team were mirrored by my friends working in software development. In that sphere, there were at least two local firms trying to develop apps to assist in test notification, contact tracing, and coordination of quarantine services. They, too, faced chilly receptions from the state government. The net result was that despite the pandemic ravaging the economy for over a year, Hawai'i developed little useful infrastructure in its private sector to help mitigate the impact of the crisis, or a future one.

This is a side story to my larger tale, but it's an important one. It echoes the problems I experienced on the medical side, but from the perspective of the business community. When I spoke with Sullivan about his experience, he was clear that the SARS-CoV-2 LFA is only a small part of what Oceanit does. Their interest in it arose out of a desire to help the state respond effectively to the pandemic. Wasn't this exactly what their counterparts in Korea had done? But Sullivan's primary interest is not in diagnostic testing. It's in building a more resilient and diversified economy, so that Hawai'i is not forever dependent on a single industry. It's the idea of hiring bright young people, and allowing them to innovate in a homegrown tech industry, that really excites him. This gets at something much deeper than testing, or even the pandemic. It's the future of Hawai'i—and the opportunities afforded its most talented residents—that's at stake.

Building new industries in Hawai'i was never likely to happen without struggle, and in the early summer, I had more concrete concerns. After the first wave receded, our local hui of doctors, epidemiologists, and economists met to decide its focus. While still frustrated by the Department of Health, we felt a growing ability to guide the state's conversation. David and I met regularly with Mayor Caldwell. David was also in touch with Lt. Gov. Josh Green, not to mention several movers in the business community. I was plugged into Queen's through the clinical trials group and, more importantly, years of good relationships with doctors and nurses. Chad Meyer was in contact with the authorities on Maui. Jerry Murphy still sat on HI-EMA, and though they ignored his good advice, he had insight into their deliberations. Building up this fund of influence in such a short time was a new experience for me. But in the end, what I cared about was winning, and winning meant keeping the virus from overrunning the Islands. We spent any influence we accrued on the goal of beating the disease.

Our initial effort centered on a couple of public letters addressed to Governor Ige. Jerry penned the first, and its focus was on shoring up relevant public health infrastructure. Without being too directly critical of the DOH, he argued that Hawaiʻi needed to enhance the effort to test, trace, and isolate all cases, and that the current infrastructure would be insufficient. The hui shared the letter with the mayors and the press, and it garnered over a hundred signatures from physicians. The governor didn't respond directly, but Caldwell pushed Jerry's points hard, and we felt some satisfaction when the DOH announced a partnership with University of Hawaiʻi, operating out of multiple sites, to train three hundred new contact tracers.

The elephant in the room, however, was tourism. There was constant chatter in the media, as well as government circles, about reopening the hospitality industry. This was the economic engine of the state, and as long as the state froze it, Hawaiʻi would be locked in severe recession. I was alarmed when, during one mayor's advisory committee discussion, the DOH shared their thinking on the subject. They expected the fourteen-day travel quarantine to be lifted. The DOH was against testing travelers, though they supported the quarantine for visitors. In one particularly sharp e-mail, they asserted the city "doesn't have jurisdiction" to deal with tourism. I fired off an appropriate response, but it was clear the medical community needed to tackle this before inertia alone drove the state towards a thoughtless lowering of its defenses.

After discussion with the hui, and in particular input from DeWolfe Miller, Tim Brown, and Sumner La Croix, I wrote the second letter to the governor. This reinforced Jerry's points about the public health infrastructure, but I focused particular attention on the screening of travelers. Based on modeling done by the University of Hawaiʻi Economic Research Organization (UHERO), we recommended pretravel testing for all visitors, as well as temperature and symptom screening at the airport. We estimated this would eliminate close to 80 percent of infections, as opposed to less than 50 percent if we relied purely on symptom screening.

The public letter (reproduced in the Backstory) and the UHERO report came out as a pair, the advocacy effort supporting (and relying on) the work done by the UH team.

In retrospect, reliance on a one-test system was overoptimistic, and a two-test system (before travel and after arrival) soon became standard for islands that valued border control. Serial testing, along the lines advocated by Mina and Bedford, also became the standard for COVID-free "bubbles" like the one built by the National Basketball Association. People don't shed the virus immediately after becoming infected, and some people get infected after their test and before their flight. The quality of administration of a test done before boarding an airplane is also variable. For these reasons, a single test will miss some infected travelers.

I wasn't married to one test. David and I preferred two, but we knew the state government was set against testing locally, and proposing a two-step scheme would have been immediately rejected. This is important to keep in mind, as later on, people were unhappy that our letter hadn't insisted on two tests from the very start. This was an expectation for which we could not get consensus even internally, let alone outside the medical community. I wanted the state to accept the concept that testing was required, because the alternative in June was nothing.

But I was happy to see that as soon as the hui released the letter, a loud chorus of people from all over the Islands demanded a second test. One such group was HI-COVID, an alliance of healthcare workers organized by Dayna Moore and based mostly on Maui. Another group on Kauaʻi, organizing around JoAnn Yukimura, the former mayor, also wanted more stringent test-based border control. I met with both groups, and recognizing like-minded people, I joined the rebels.

In the meantime, the second letter collected over four hundred signatures from healthcare workers. Daniel Ross from the nurse's union was particularly helpful. Having the nurses speak in unison on a public health measure supercharged the effort. We delivered the letter to Governor Ige and the mayor, as well as the press. Soon afterwards I did an interview on Hawaii Public Radio (HPR), in which I called the temperature screens at arrival terminals "airport theatre," and called for the governor to protect the health of the Islands by setting up a test-based system. In an interview that aired just after my own, HPR peppered the governor with questions about the border, and he maneuvered to respond to my points.

It was an honor to be able to voice the feelings of a great number of healthcare workers, particularly on a matter of such consequence. That evening, as I listened to the governor speak, I reflected on political power. It's an intangible substance. Like a rumor, it comes and goes without sticking to anyone. The people in authority, who had been blocking our efforts, suddenly lacked it. And I, speaking as a doctor on behalf of my patients and my town, for one fleeting moment possessed it. I won't deny the feeling of exhilaration I experienced at the realization my words were having the desired impact. I slept soundly, knowing I had landed a solid blow.

In this effort, we had no direct collaboration with Lt. Gov. Josh Green, but the grassroots push complemented his internal battle against the DOH. Soon, Ige accepted testing as inevitable, and he placed Green in charge of drawing up the protocol. This would soon become the Safe Travels program, and it would be based on a pretravel test combined with symptomatic screening. But many questions remained. Who would help Green write the protocol? What mechanism would be put in place for quarantine enforcement? What process would we use for critical infrastructure workers? What about post-arrival testing? It soon became apparent that the business community had the main seat at the table, and that these questions would fester.

This disappointment didn't dissuade me much. The hui had made real progress in pushing the state towards a test-based border control. One test wasn't good enough in itself, but I thought purity was an overrated virtue. A pretravel test, paired with symptom screening, was far better than nothing. I was confident it would save lives. And during a pandemic, the politicians ignore clinicians and epidemiologists at their peril. The growing chorus around me, the voices of hundreds of bright people demanding an even more effective border and travel system, gave me confidence to continue to push for the vision of a COVID-free Hawaiʻi. ☙

Chapter Ten

THE SECOND WAVE

JULY 31, 2020

2,172
HAWAIʻI

4,388,566	17,105,266
UNITED STATES	WORLD

COVID-19 cases (data sources: World Health Organization and Hawaii Department of Health)

Conspiratorial thinking and denial of many kinds had been part of the ethos since the spring, but in the first two months of the epidemic it was possible to overlook the signs of division. When the disease was new, few countries did well with it, and political quarrels felt less salient. It was the progressive states, especially New York, that had the biggest epidemics. These were paralleled by equally large epidemics in Western Europe, which overwhelmed the socialist healthcare systems in Italy, Spain, and other countries. The United States had shut down, and though resistance to public health measures was evident, in April and May, experts had the upper hand in policy discussions.

But by the summer, the epidemic in the United States began to diverge sharply from Europe. Most countries in Europe sustained long and restrictive lockdowns, relying on generous welfare benefits to keep their citizens fed and housed. In the United States, there was tremendous pressure to reopen the economy. This was both economic and ideological. Welfare benefits paled in comparison to Europe, and people needed to work. Wraparound services to keep people safely quarantined simply did not exist in most places. But there was also a backlash to government dictates, drawing on the libertarian instincts at the root of the American culture. Under normal circumstances, this is a healthy part of American life, but during the pandemic, when common action was more critical than ever before, conspiracists preyed effectively on the distrust of authority. A stronger leadership culture may have maintained discipline and cohesion. But in 2020, the United States lacked leaders capable of inspiring self-sacrifice, or even cooperation.

Shutdowns in the South and West ended early, and high-risk activities like bars resumed long before case counts were sufficiently low to prevent a rebound. Republican politicians, following the president's lead, downplayed the danger of the virus. The result was that Europe's

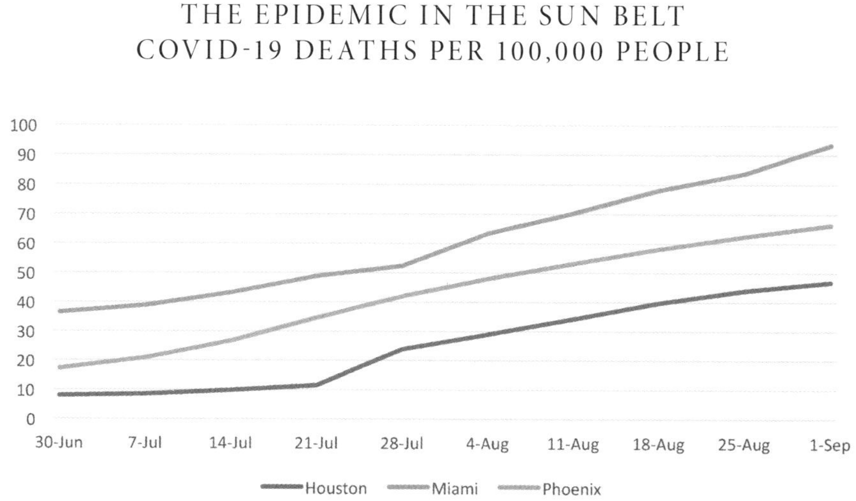

Figure 11.1 Data Source—USA Facts, CDC. Graph by author

epidemic curve plunged towards zero, while America's entered a plateau. Then in June and July, to the surprise of many who expected a respite until winter, cases began to spike as large outbreaks gripped the Sun Belt states. ICUs in Florida, Texas, and Arizona began to fill, and the rising case counts shattered any illusion that normal life could resume, or that the weather was sufficient cause for optimism.

In Canada, where the level of social cohesion and welfare was higher, the epidemic followed a much more European trajectory. Anyone arguing for the exceptionalism of the American system suddenly had to confront the obvious failure of the country relative to its peers.

There are moments in history when the psychology of power shifts in subtle but profound ways, and this was one of them. An epidemic that arose in China had spread to the world. The Chinese authorities contained the disease with remarkable efficiency. The United States, long-perceived as the bulwark against Chinese coercion, lacked even basic logistical competence. By the summer, the country was staggering into a second wave, highlighted publicly by bitter squabbling and assertions of magical thinking. Nothing in the past century was more humiliating to the idea of American prestige. The country appeared to be manifestly past its prime.

Hawai'i benefited from a lower baseline of disease, in large part due to the shutdown during April and May and the state's ability to control its border. But much of the dysfunction that crippled the Mainland existed here as well, and the state was soon to pay the price for it.

In June, Hawai'i experienced the beginning of a sustained increase in the daily case numbers. The problem was most pronounced on O'ahu, where it became common to see large gatherings of people congregating under beach tents, or in the stands at outdoor youth sporting events. It wasn't clear how much this contributed to transmission, and that was itself part of the problem. The state provided little reliable data on where transmission was happening. The DOH either didn't have it or wouldn't share it. In general, outdoor activities were safe, but with large gatherings there were no guarantees, and the large crowds sent a message of false reassurance that life was back to normal.

Even more concerning were reports of cases in the Pacific Islander community, many of whom lived in public housing complexes in Kalihi Valley. This was the densest part of Honolulu, with multigenerational families often crowded into small apartments. It was also David Derauf's core constituency, and as his patients became ill, he became increasingly frustrated. He had warned about precisely this occurrence back in March, during some of our first meetings with state and city. What had been put in place to protect these people? There was no asymptomatic screening. There was little support for people to stay home from work while ill. Effective quarantine often wasn't possible at home given their living situations, and the state had blocked every attempt to set up an efficient hotel quarantine scheme. David watched in horror as the epidemic took off in his neighborhood, and I often found him in high dudgeon when speaking with city or state officials.

By late summer, the spread of disease within the Pacific Islander community became so severe that it behaved, in the words of DeWolfe Miller, as an "epidemic within the epidemic." One aspect of this sub-epidemic was that it spared Native Hawaiians, who had case rates similar to Caucasians. But amongst immigrants from other Pacific islands, the epidemic was especially cruel. DeWolfe and his colleagues tabulated this data and produced a graph in the *International Journal of Infectious Diseases.*

DeWolfe worked with Josie Howard of We Are Oceania, an organization representing Pacific Islanders, and improvements in mask use eventually made progress in squashing the sub-epidemic. Most of this success happened in the background, without much attention from the press, and despite the early neglect of the health authorities. But without the accomplishment of the Pacific Islanders, the broader pandemic control effort in Hawai'i would have been doomed. Their achievement, painfully won, would not reach maturity until fall and winter.

The summer surge in Hawai'i iced the plan to reopen tourism, as testing resources were consumed trying to contain the local epidemic. National shortages put testing under so much strain that DLS had to again, temporarily, restrict access. This made it impractical to test arriving passengers, and shortages of tests on the Mainland made it hard to implement pretravel screening. But the situation also made Hawai'i a

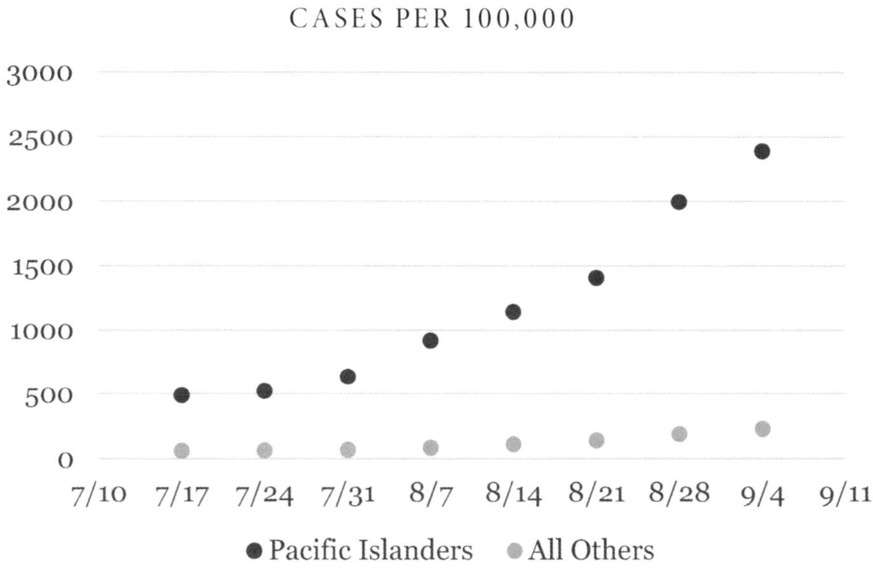

Figure 10.2 – Data Source DeWolfe Miller et al. *(graph adapted with permission from the authors). Case rates per hundred thousand (vertical axis) in Pacific Islanders (dark dots) were ten times higher than in all other ethnicities (light dots) in Hawai'i.*

less attractive destination for travelers. The state's brand as a disease-free location was irreparably damaged as the case numbers exploded.

One problem for Mayor Caldwell was his reliance on the state for core public health functions. He commanded no city department of health, and he was told repeatedly that the state contact tracing operation was adequately staffed. This never corresponded with what I saw on the ground. Despite the agreement between the DOH and University of Hawai'i to train contact tracers, a source of pride for our hui after our first letter, there was no evidence that more tracers were working. Many patients weren't contacted for several days after their diagnosis, and it was difficult to get anyone a hotel room. DOH officers continued to not test asymptomatic family members.

It was the subject of the failed public health effort that formed the basis of my one direct interaction with Governor David Ige. JoAnn Yukimura arranged a meeting with the governor to discuss a variety of topics, from test-based border control to the epidemic in Kalihi. She graciously invited me to participate. The meeting occurred August 4, and it included numerous people affiliated with the Kauaʻi working group. Michael Schwartz, a professor at the University of Washington, gave the governor a detailed breakdown of the scientific concerns with a single, pretravel test. David Derauf spoke about the outbreak in Kalihi and the lack of disease control in public housing. Kapono Chong-Hanssen discussed the experience of Native Hawaiians, and he advocated for creating a "*kīpuka,*" a COVID-free state safe for the residents.

Amongst this talented company, I didn't say much. Time was in short supply, and I thought it best to allow the others to make their case. But when the governor volunteered his view that all close contacts of infected patients should be tested, I made my single interjection. I pointed out that not only was testing of asymptomatic contacts not happening, but that even before the second surge of cases, the DOH was refusing to perform this function. The governor asked me why this was not happening. This was his only question in the meeting. I responded that I was told by the DOH it wasn't necessary. The governor looked down at his notepad and wrote a few words.

I was impressed by this exchange, and others were, too. We discussed it in the debriefing. The governor had the appearance in that moment of encountering a reality different than the one that had been presented to him by official sources. He clearly wasn't happy about it. But it's also notable what did not happen. He didn't say, "We're going to fix this." And looking back on it, he didn't seem terribly surprised either to hear that some fact presented to him by his subordinates was being directly contradicted by a clinical doctor.

Mayor Caldwell's response to the morass at the state level was to expand the county's testing program, as well as to pay for isolation and quarantine rooms. This was good, but it was no substitute for a comprehensive strategy between city and state. Furthermore, the qualities that made the mayor likable and empathetic did not serve him as well in the face of intense, often angry, pressure from suffering businesses. Once the city began to open up, it proved impossible for the mayor to proceed slowly and in stages. During the eight weeks spanning May 6 to July 2, Caldwell issued nine emergency orders, as well as a guidance bulletin and a supplemental proclamation. I began hearing credible rumors of packed crowds at bars and in nightclubs. Church services with large congregations were allowed, as long as there was a pretense of physical spacing. In reality, physical distancing was gone, and the rules issued were so complex that the mayor's own team struggled to keep up with them. Most importantly, the reopening messaging failed to engage the leaders of the Pacific Islander community. A few funerals in that community became superspreader events that put disease control beyond the reach of any authority.

In conversations about the various county restrictions, it's important to distinguish between honest disagreements and dishonest ones. Many people, including those in the fields of infectious diseases and public health, did not agree on the timing, severity, or duration of restrictions. Pandemics drag on for months, if not years, and the effort to counter a pandemic is something like a marathon. Furthermore, the science of virus transmission was still being worked out during the first several months of 2020, as were the most appropriate mechanisms of disease control. It would have been unreasonable to expect perfect consistency or agreement amongst even the most knowledgeable people. I thought that intelligent and well-intentioned people could disagree about the details.

However, there was another element that had entered the equation across the United States, a vocal minority that spread disinformation about the pandemic with a kind of ideological fervor. These people tended to be anti-vaccine, anti–mask wearing, and anti–social distancing. They were paranoid about authority and contemptuous of expertise. They reminded me of religious fundamentalists I had spoken with in travels to the Middle East. They had a predetermined and suspicious worldview, matched with a disregard for the facts.

As early as April or May, it was clear this faction wasn't just living in its own reality, but was also perfectly willing to get other people killed. I was a tolerant person on matters of politics, but this was a different matter. Arguing with this element was a kind of asymmetric warfare, because they didn't play by the same rules of truth seeking and mutual aid that most people adopted as a starting assumption. The supply of protective equipment at Queen's was limited, and I recognized that my colleagues and I were at increased risk of injury and death because of this new extremism. I thought Honolulu would have to choose what attitudes it would not put up with. That was not a hard choice for me. I valued the lives of nurses and doctors over the offended sensibilities of political fanatics. I thought they should be forced to suffer the hell of a competent pandemic response.

This came up in the mayor's meetings, in which "the knuckleheads" were an occasional theme. My advice to Caldwell was fairly simple. It was something like, "Crush them, and let everyone see you crushing them." The crushing was of course metaphorical. I wanted to see the most important rules—like the entry quarantine—enforced unapologetically. For the vast majority of people trying to do the right thing, I thought it was necessary for morale to see the mayor protecting the public. There was nothing to be gained by appeasing the extremists, because they despised our efforts on principle.

Not everyone agreed with my tone. The issue of "shame" often came up in a negative context. Even doctors who tried to promote mask wearing made frequent reference to "mask shaming," arguing that being heavy-handed only caused people to dig in further. The details matter, and each conversation is unique. I agreed that confrontation was rarely helpful. But as a general observation, I never bought into the notion that shaming people was something to be sorry about. Shame, after all, is a sense of pain at the knowledge of one's wrongdoing. As an emotional response, it is socially evolved and highly useful. There's no violence in shame, or even the threat of violence. It relies implicitly on a person's sense of right and wrong, as well as one's obligations to the community. A person who puts his elderly neighbor at risk of death because he is too self-absorbed to wear a mask, or to curtail his nightclub habit, should feel ashamed. Any other emotion in that context is inappropriate, even antisocial. It's for this reason that the appeals to discourage shaming struck me as timid. A number of jurisdictions would have done well by encouraging a healthy sense of shame, rather than coddling their sociopaths.

Such was my mood early on. But by June and July I thought that the majority of frustrations, at least in Honolulu, were the honest kind. City residents questioned rules that violated best public health practices. The closure of public beaches, intended to break up large crowds, angered thousands of people who had previously supported the city's efforts. The order was in contrast to rules that allowed many indoor businesses to continue to function, and it created the perception that the city was ignoring the science and picking winners amongst the business community. Parents who had been home for months with toddlers were not allowed to access parks, while other adults went shopping. The perception of corrupt intent was nearly fatal. In my own social circle, this was the only time I encountered bitterness directed personally towards the mayor.

The thinking behind these decisions was not malevolent, but it was still unflattering to the city's effort. The medical advisory group emphasized repeatedly that outdoor activity was safer than indoor, but most of us felt it reasonable to break up large crowds. I wanted crowd size to determine police behavior, and I hoped for gentle reminders rather than citations. The mayor agreed, but the police insisted on a more simple "open or closed" formulation for parks and beaches. I was not privy to the internal discussion between mayor and police. Later, Caldwell told me that the police expressed concern that they couldn't break up large crowds without violence. There was racial and economic disparity in who made most frequent use of Hawai'i beaches. In the midst of the Black Lives Matter protests, the police were sensitive to any charge of discriminatory enforcement. I wonder if there was a subtle middle finger being extended to a government populated by political liberals, who had embraced an anti-police movement only to find themselves in urgent need of police cooperation. The mayor, in turn, opted for "all" rather than "nothing," and he closed the beaches.

The city needed the police to do two core functions to make

its pandemic response effective. It needed help enforcing the entry quarantine, and it needed help breaking up large gatherings. It needed them to do both those tasks with tact and efficiency, in addition to continuing their regular police duties, which put them under strain given the economic conditions. These were big asks. In fact, there was no agency, except the Department of Health, that was more important to Honolulu's success. Unlike the DOH, the police were a city agency. The mayor certainly lavished them with resources, including new equipment and funding for overtime. But their unwillingness to grapple with crowds sensibly, even while providing a hundred other necessary functions, undermined public confidence in the entire disease control effort.

The city should have demanded more of the police, and it should have supported them through any resulting criticism. As it played out, the mayor hemorrhaged much of the goodwill he had accumulated in the spring, and the draconian enforcement carried out by the police further undermined both his status and theirs. Civil Beat, in particular, made a sport of writing articles about police funding and corruption. When the cops busted the US surgeon general for walking harmlessly on a beach during a visit hastily arranged to help Oʻahu with its still surging case counts, the rules became a farce.

In July, the infectious diseases division at Queen's resurrected the COVID call schedule. I went back on service, and we were busier than we had been in April. The internal medicine doctor the week I was on was Lester Morehead. Lester is a former military doc from Louisiana who had served in both Iraq and Afghanistan. He is also an unredeemable smart-ass. Queen's administration was weary of him, as he had a talent for pointing out leadership shortcomings. I often teased him that he agreed to get shot at because it gave him the right to bitch, and that was his true priority in life. But I also thought he was one of the most skilled internists I ever worked with. He was the perfect doctor for COVID, quick on his feet and unafraid. Now we were on service together, getting shot at by a virus, and we indulged in a nonstop banter of dark humor. I'm not sure how the nurses took us. The ward was filling up with patients, and the two of us were acting completely unserious. But this concealed a deeper anxiety. We both subscribed to the notion that in a frightening situation the best tactic was to talk a lot of trash.

The medical care during this second wave was better. The hospital was no longer desperately short of protective gear, which made it easier to round. Months of published literature had made me more attuned to complications of the virus, including thrombotic events and secondary infections. I made use of the antiviral drug remdesivir, which I gave to anyone who came in with an oxygen requirement. There was a protocol for convalescent plasma. Sicker patients received the steroid dexamethasone, based on a mortality benefit shown in a large UK trial. The COVID medical advisory group, working through Todd Seto's clinical trials team, had also begun a trial for an IL-6 inhibitor (another immune modulatory drug) to be used in critically ill patients suffering from "cytokine storm," or badly hyperactive immune responses. As randomized trial data became available, it became clear that not all of these treatments worked. But the net result was that the local mortality rate dropped even as cases surged past the April peak.

It's worth reflecting on this rapid evolution of medical care. In just a few months, the hospital had jettisoned hydroxychloroquine (the subject of much angst early on) in favor of a panoply of new treatments. These, in turn, were often based on limited data, and as new trials came out, standards of care were constantly upended. It was common to practice in a particular way one week, only to go 180 degrees in the opposite direction the next. One example of this was dexamethasone. Prior to the UK RECOVERY trial, many treatment algorithms (which were prepared and updated by academic medical centers) recommended against using steroids. That was based, in part, on bad experiences with steroids in influenza, which in the spring was treated as analogous to SARS-CoV-2. However, as more data emerged on the importance of inflammation in the COVID disease process, things began to change, and when clinical trial data showed a mortality benefit to steroids, that became the standard of care. I remember my sense of whiplash when I realized I would be prescribing, rather than discouraging, steroids.

Conspiracists made use of these sudden changes in recommendations to create doubt about the value of scientific expertise. But there was always an important difference between changing direction based on science, and changing direction in order to placate politics. My problem with the CDC during COVID was they too often did the latter. That created a legitimate basis for distrust. But the problem wasn't the change, it was the politics. The beauty of the scientific process is that its thinking changes based on evidence. When a more successful paradigm emerges, it obligates doctors to update their thinking. This is a strength, not a weakness, of allopathic medicine, and there is no other medical paradigm in the world that matches this virtue. The country would have prospered far better during 2020 if its millions of ideologues and zealots could do the same.

In this fitful way, treatments improved from spring to summer, but I was deflated by the lack of a truly excellent antiviral medicine. Remdesivir never showed a mortality benefit, and additional data from the World Health Organization revealed even its limited claims of efficacy to be suspect. Convalescent plasma, another idea taken from the history of influenza treatments, also faded in importance as numerous studies showed no benefit. As an infectious diseases doctor, I disliked the idea of using immune suppressants to fight a viral infection. I wanted a sword to slay the virus. One explanation for the failure to find a good drug was the timing of the illness. People became sick with SARS-CoV-2, but the disease moved slowly, and they often didn't present to the hospital until a week or more into the illness. By that time, doctors were seeing the immune system's inflammatory cascade, and the resultant respiratory failure. This was the sequelae of the infection, not the phase of direct viral invasion. An oral antiviral given to an outpatient earlier in the illness would have offered a better prospect of success. But in the summer of 2020, such drugs weren't available.

I felt fully engaged during my service week with Lester Morehead, and I would have been happy to continue in that role. But by July I was on my way out of Honolulu. I had resumed my visits to the Big Island, where I had a growing number of patients in Waimea. It wasn't attractive to do a lot of back-and-forth air travel during the pandemic. Layla was a teacher, and both her job and my children's school were halted by the pandemic.

The kids were home, and I thought it better to get them out of the city. I wanted them to have room to play, fresh air, and new adventures to look forward to. We had made the decision to move my practice to Queen's North Hawai'i during the summer and to school the kids from home the following year. In my nonwork hours, my mind drifted to thoughts of renovating the old farmhouse, and I thought I would do well to get a shepherd dog.

But those dreams had become plans during May, when things were quiet. I was surprised, and in truth hurt, to realize I would be leaving Honolulu during a premature surge of cases. I need not have fretted. The Big Island was short of doctors, and there would soon be virus in the country. ☙

Chapter Eleven

CHANGES IN COMMAND

AUGUST 31, 2020

8,603

HAWAI‘I

5,855,521	24,854,140
UNITED STATES	WORLD

COVID-19 cases (data sources: World Health Organization and Hawaii Department of Health)

The second wave peaked not long after my move, and it exceeded anything Hawai‘i experienced in the spring. At its height, the state averaged three hundred cases per day, the vast majority on O‘ahu, an attack rate that was ten times worse than the April surge. And while the hospitals were much better prepared, the scale of the assault badly strained resources. Queen's quickly filled up with COVID, peaking at just over a hundred admissions. Most patients resided on the medical wards, but the virus also filled the medical intensive care unit and spilled over into neighboring ICUs. PPE recycling resumed, and the strain on remdesivir supply became too high to use it on every admission. This kind of care rationing alarmed me, as it suggested that the virus was still capable of overwhelming the state's infrastructure. The greatest strain was on individuals. Doctors and nurses on the COVID units worked in difficult circumstances, and not everyone handled it as well as Lester Morehead. I was particularly concerned about the potential for hospital clusters. These could take out healthcare workers directly, leaving the hospitals understaffed at the worst moment. This was the scenario that would lead to much higher mortality rates. I worried that if Oʻahu did not interrupt transmission, the system would break.

This is what Oʻahu looked like with three hundred cases per day, the majority occurring in vulnerable subpopulations. After discussing the situation with friends in our hui, David and I concluded that the island was nowhere close to herd immunity. If transmission became more widespread, we could see more than one thousand cases per day, and the strain that would place on resources would be inconceivable.

I reached out to the mayor and arranged for him to visit Queen's. In doing so, I alerted a few of my medicine colleagues, including Ryan Honda. Honda had been involved in leadership of the hospitalist group for years, and he worked as one of the COVID physicians. On big problems, we always found a way to come together. This was no exception. Honda arranged to greet the mayor, and most importantly from my perspective, ensured that he could speak with COVID unit doctors and nurses. It was important that he not be whisked off into a conference room or distracted by a PowerPoint presentation. I wanted him to look a nurse in the eye.

Kirk Caldwell arrived, accompanied by Libby Char, and although Queen's hastily organized an administrative greeting, he spent most of his time with the docs and nurses. The mayor had a talent for listening, and he made a good impression. He expressed his concerns transparently to the staff and asked them about a second shutdown. As with any group, opinions were mixed, but he saw the weariness on their faces. He left Queen's with a firmer sense of what he wanted to do, and the following week he announced the second shutdown of Honolulu.

I expected a backlash against any stay-at-home order. This was the second time Oʻahu was going through the trauma of a freeze of its economic and cultural life. The unity of purpose that had graced the effort to control the disease in April was now absent. Large numbers of people were reading propaganda online, and some of the major news networks were spreading it. There were also good reasons to distrust the government. The state had failed to erect a competent public health response, wasting months of time when cases were low, and the local epidemic exploded despite a continued closure of tourism. People had sacrificed, and for what? The governor complimented his DOH, insisting they had "one of the best" contact tracing efforts in the country. This lack of attachment to reality was demoralizing.

The mayor had fared better, but just barely. The series of confusing orders restricting business and social activity had angered residents but failed to prevent transmission. The mayor was trying to navigate numerous pressures. But I was sure that during the pandemic he would have done best politically by walloping the virus and making everyone else adjust.

How easy it is, from the outside, to see the fault in another man's work. But how difficult it is to walk his path! Coronavirus was a killer of towns across America, and no government handled it perfectly. Honolulu had a mayor who believed it was his duty to fight the disease, and he was willing to ruin his own prospects to beat it. As a doctor, I was grateful to find someone in Hawaiʻi's government who felt this way. History will treat him more gently than a few heated opinion polls in 2020.

I tried to help the mayor through this excruciating period by focusing on action that the city could undertake to break the second wave and prevent a third. In a letter dated August 21, I advised:

> There are numerous problems with allowing uncontrolled transmission to continue on Oʻahu, a situation that is likely if we don't alter course.
>
> 1) Epidemiology studies from other countries suggest that most transmission occurs indoors during work and recreation, and we have left many of these venues open.
>
> 2) A partial shutdown (*i.e.*, the scalpel) approach would be preferable if we

could make that work. But for it to work we have to be able to target it, and we likely needed to do that several weeks ago. We're now seeing widespread and largely untraced transmission, which makes piecemeal interventions less likely to succeed.

3) We don't understand the long-term sequelae of COVID. There are reports of cardiac and neurocognitive damage. If we allow this to run through the population we may be left with tens of thousands of people who suffer from chronic health problems. This is a separate problem from the expected ICU surge and mortality event.

4) By giving up on disease containment we're also making it impossible for Hawai'i's economic and education institutions to recover. Schools will be closed. This will warp the experience of children and take their working parents out of the labor force. Hawai'i will not recover as a travel destination, because people won't want to come here. Small businesses will be paralyzed as they lose customers. Workers will become sick or stay home to care for children. We'll suffer many of the same economic impacts of a shutdown, but they will be piled on top of a healthcare crisis.

There's no winning without containing the disease. We need a more coherent strategy that the population can understand and police can enforce. We need to catch up in regards to testing, tracing, and isolation. We need to get infected people out of crowded housing and into hotel rooms, and provide services to support them until case numbers drop off. Reopening schools should be an early priority. Lifting the interisland quarantine should also be a priority. These things don't happen with uncontrolled transmission.

To make any shutdown and reopening stick, we need to correct the deficiencies in our last reopening. This means building useful public health infrastructure. The counties and private enterprise should take the lead here, with federal help if needed. We punted to the state government in April and May, and the results speak for themselves.

Direct and honest communication with the public will be critical to make any containment strategy work. We should expect anger after months of failed state policies. We can't just offer advice on what's good behavior. We need to be honest about what has failed in the response so far and what we're doing to fix it. And we need to hold ourselves accountable for fixing it.

I was more specific in another letter, dated August 26, in which I outlined the key elements of test-trace-isolate-support, suggesting how these could be integrated by a partnership between the city and private enterprise:

> There are several measures the city can take during this shutdown to defeat the virus. I hope to highlight potential pitfalls so that we can avoid the mistakes that doomed previous efforts.
>
> In order for the public health response to work it needs to bundle into a coherent whole. The biggest mistake is allowing institutional turf to fragment the response. The interventions must all swim together, or we drown.
>
> 1) Target tests where COVID-19 is. To get the most out of testing we need to target it at the most impacted communities. This should include a push to get every close contact of a new case tested within twenty-four hours and into contact tracing. The new CDC statement that de-emphasizes testing close contacts will get people killed, and you should ignore it. Testing should also focus on Kalihi, public housing, and other high-transmission venues. Testing for city employees and frontline workers should happen, but not instead of communities that are suffering uncontrolled disease. Testing thousands won't help us if we miss the disease.
>
> 2) Stand up contact tracing. This needs to happen at scale, and we would be fools to rely on the DOH. The model proposed by Hiro Toiya, where contact tracers are paid by the city and assigned to health centers, is a good start. I favor having an additional group of tracers that form a reserve and can be used for patients who are not clients of any particular health center or when a health center needs additional support. The goal is to have every new case traced within twenty-four hours, regardless of providing doctor.
>
> 3) Provide hotels and wraparound care. These need to be expanded, linked closely with testing, and made available to anyone who needs them. Expect a need for over a thousand hotel rooms in order to appropriately decongest crowded housing. Ancillary services, including medical check-ins, COVID-safe transportation, food delivery, and financial assistance for people missing work should be provided. Any failure in the wraparound service will cause the entire structure of test-trace-isolate to crumble.
>
> To summarize, the response begins with testing. But a positive result prompts a series of interactions with the county that lead to deployment of additional resources. The patient's family must be immediately tested. During that time a contact tracer should take a history and initiate any further needed testing and

> quarantine. That effort integrates with the hotel and transport teams, who place anyone that needs a room. Tracing links to wraparound services, including medical check-ins, food delivery, and financial assistance.
>
> This is a big lift, and it's not fair that the task has fallen to the city. But the virus doesn't care about what's fair. It will spread relentlessly and paralyze the island until we thwart it. The good news is that many people with relevant expertise exist to help, and they are eager to become involved. The state's inability to bring all our talent to bear was a failure of political imagination, and we are now in a crisis that you have a unique and historical opportunity to correct. It's the integration of thousands of people, working to serve their community, that will save O'ahu. The leadership of your team is what makes that possible and glues the effort together.

In these communications I appealed to the mayor's sense of history, and to the duties thrust upon him by the failure of the state effort. I knew the mayor never wanted to have to confront such terrible problems alone, and given the structure of Hawai'i's government, he never should have had to. But I also knew he would relish the opportunity to solve problems that others had shied away from. He received these messages with grace, and as the city went into the second lockdown, Caldwell's efforts to scale up testing, contact tracing, and hotel room isolation showed a growing and effective urgency.

It was during this time of tumult, in the latter half of August and the beginning of September, that Hawai'i effected changes in leadership that would prove decisive for the coming months. I had a small and uncomfortable role in this, due to my presence on social media. Over the course of the year, my Facebook account had become a local forum for discussing Hawai'i's pandemic response. In mid-August I composed a post taking the state to task for the failure to increase testing, contact tracing, and quarantine. This was the most public I had been in my criticism of government officials. I took no joy in voicing the displeasure of healthcare professionals. I would have preferred that Hawai'i's leaders did well, and I could help explain the necessity of their actions. I had, in numerous conversations, tried to address failures in private. But it had become clear that this was getting no response, and now people were dying as a result. Even worse, the Health Department was doubling down. As the case count rose, the department insisted it couldn't share more information on where cases occurred, because of privacy concerns.

For me, this was the final straw. I have found that in medicine the appeal to privacy is often the refuge of scoundrels. The federal privacy law, known as the Health Information Portability and Accountability Act (HIPPAA), is frequently used as a tool of obstruction. Through time-consuming paperwork requirements, intended to ward off legal penalties, HIPPAA has contributed to the fragmentation of record keeping that makes care in American hospitals disjointed. People who don't want to cooperate with others love HIPPAA. But to invoke it during a public health crisis showed not just bad judgment, but suspect intentions. The state was failing, and it desperately needed a better working relationship between physicians and government. There were some tactical considerations informing my timing as well. Having recently moved to the Big Island, I was in a better position to voice the concerns of my colleagues, many of whom were still enmeshed with state authorities professionally and dependent on them for care of patients. But I felt confident that once my fingers struck the keys, I would be voicing the pent-up frustration of a great number of doctors who had held their tongues too long.

I posted my criticism on Facebook August 14, and within a couple days, hundreds of people shared the link. I received a call from Kirk Caldwell, who asked me if he could forward it to the *Star-Advertiser.* Given the newfound success of my online efforts, I thought his attachment to print media somewhat old fashioned. But of course, he was correct to point out that many thousands of people in the state, particularly in the older generation, still relied on the newspaper. These were precisely the people whose opinion the governor cared about. Facebook had given me a bigger megaphone than I had ever expected, but it was a fickle medium, subject to endless disinformation.

I readily agreed to Caldwell's suggestion. This was the longest conversation I had with the mayor. He laughed at the coqui frogs calling in the background at my new home, and I noted that he seemed amused, rather than offended, that I had relocated from Honolulu to the country.

The mayor himself had grown up in this rural part of Hawai'i, and he spent some time reminiscing with me about his childhood home in Reeds Island.

The op-ed ran Sunday the 23rd in the *Star-Advertiser*, and it was referenced by a *New York Times* article on Hawai'i's sputtering pandemic response. My in-box filled with comments, mostly supportive, but there was notable silence from a few quarters. I understood all too well that in calling out the state's failure I had made some enemies, and my own access to powerful people might be curtailed. But I also understood that in a mortal struggle, which the state was certainly facing, truth was the only path to safety. I felt I had no alternative, and I didn't worry overmuch about discomfiting a few officials.

By now, things were rapidly deteriorating for the DOH leadership. In early August, Sarah Park appeared before the Senate COVID committee. Unsatisfied with her testimony, state legislators staged an unannounced inspection of DOH headquarters. During this impromptu visit, the senators discovered an understaffed and overwhelmed contact tracing effort. My perception that the DOH wasn't doing contact tracing turned out to be incorrect. In fact, there were extremely dedicated workers attempting to keep up with a deluge of cases. They were working long hours, coming in on weekends, and taking on tasks beyond the work of contact investigation. But their number was closer to ten than a hundred, and the three hundred UH contact tracers were never brought in.

The site visit corresponded with a government employee union complaint that the state had not adequately staffed the operation. Subsequent reporting in Civil Beat and elsewhere confirmed no more than a few dozen contact tracers. The official number was over a hundred, itself felt to be too low. Where were the missing tracers? How had the federal money for that program been spent?

Some of the confusion regarding the number of tracers is due to how that function is defined. The Department of Health has a division for disease investigation, and the job description of those investigators includes contact tracing. But this flexibility in assignment allowed the department to obscure how many people were directly employed and supported in the contact tracing effort.

At this time a whistleblower, a DOH virologist named Jennifer Smith, came forward with details about the contact tracing operation at DOH. Not only were they terribly understaffed, but Smith felt tracers had no support from leadership to do their jobs. The small group had no prospect of contacting or testing anyone in a timely way. Smith described a feeling of "panic" as case counts continued to rise, burying them further behind. While this deterioration of disease investigation had continued in private, the state's epidemic curve took on the appearance of a SpaceX rocket trail.

A full scandal now enveloped Governor Ige, and long-standing concerns about his leadership transformed into talk of impeachment. The governor, still not acknowledging the problems gripping his pandemic response, nonetheless felt it time to announce the retirement of the director of health. Bruce Anderson agreed to leave office on September 15. The final shove came from the department itself, where Emily Roberson, newly in charge of contact tracing, demanded clarification of her leadership chain before taking responsibility for the faltering effort. Her demand prompted the exit of Sarah Park, who was put on administrative leave. Park never returned.

In less than a month, the balance of power had shifted completely. The Department of Health, until now a powerful state institution blocking Caldwell's efforts, was reeling. The governor began working with Caldwell to create a more effective city–state partnership. My two letters arguing for an integrated disease control effort occurred in the context of this vacuum, but I didn't realize how close we were to achieving a major gain in influence at the state level. Caldwell was operating on the political plane, and he moved quickly not only to fill the public health void with city resources, but to reshape the relationship between Honolulu and the DOH.

With Anderson and Park out, a new set of personalities began to emerge at the state level. Sarah Kemble became the state's acting epidemiologist, and she quickly established a friendly and collaborative rapport with physicians. Emily Roberson had unfettered control of contact tracing, and she began to reorganize that effort. The mayor offered hundreds of contact tracers to help her staff up. With the state and city efforts finally merging, a series of private meetings commenced with the purpose of overhauling the state response. Additional changes were forthcoming. Quarantine, long stifled by the DOH's disease outbreak control division, was transferred to the behavioral health division. That put Eddie Mersereau in charge. Eddie is a guy used to dealing with complicated social problems, and he brought a more flexible mindset to the challenge. He moved quickly to expand the hotel capacity, simplify eligibility criteria, and strengthen wraparound care for isolated patients.

Most importantly, the state needed to choose a replacement for Bruce Anderson. The director of health was the top role at DOH, and the director had broad authority to set agendas and assign personnel. I had gotten so used to an inaccessible director that I almost forgot about the position. But it was at the very heart of the state's response. I became aware through private messages that Libby Char was offered the job. I contacted her immediately, and my advice was simple: "If they are offering you real authority, please take it."

Libby disliked attention, and she had deep reservations about her ability to effect positive change at the DOH. But this was an emergency, with the prospect of thousands of deaths looming. All of us who knew her felt she had the right temperament for the job. The department, and in truth the entire state government, was short on leadership. Libby brought a strong sense of personal integrity, a desire to collaborate well with bright people, and an impatience with obfuscation. Sometimes the moment chooses the woman. I thought it had chosen well, and that night I slept soundly, unbothered by the chorus of scandal in the press or the romantic troubles of the coquis outside my window. ♥

Chapter Twelve

HOLDING THE SHIELD

SEPTEMBER 30, 2020

12,453

HAWAIʻI

6,960,152	32,730,945
UNITED STATES	WORLD

COVID-19 cases (data sources: World Health Organization and Hawaii Department of Health)

The Mainland entered its third wave in the autumn. This would greatly surpass anything that came before, with cases now so widespread that the outbreak was essentially national. In September, the death count passed two hundred thousand. The president promised law and order in the cities, but with CARES Act funding running out, he offered no further aid. This was a critical factor, as much of Honolulu's ability to take on public health tasks and provide economic support to people impacted by the pandemic depended on federal aid.

On Rosh Hashanah, Supreme Court justice Ruth Bader Ginsburg died. Trump moved quickly to fill the vacancy with a choice that would please evangelical Christians. With the election only weeks away, this was a power move for a faltering president. It provided an argument for reelection that appealed to the cultural anxieties of his base, and it distracted them from the lethal failure to address the pandemic that was unfolding before them.

No one should be surprised that people who suffered on the scale that Americans suffered in 2020 had trouble dealing clearly with reality. In the final toll, there would be more than six hundred thousand deaths, most occurring at the end of 2020 and in the first few months of the new year. Those deaths occurred despite a massive, nationwide effort by the country's hospitals and intensive care units to keep people alive. They occurred despite the new therapies available, and despite harsh restrictions imposed in many cities to control transmission. Tens of millions of people became ill during these months. When death and illness are everywhere, make-believe isn't just the defense of small children. The virus was most threatening not because of the exceptional number it killed, but because of its capacity to make everyday life dangerous. It was a natural response to dissociate from this. And when the government proved incapable of controlling the epidemic, or even speaking about it honestly, it was inevitable that social cohesion would fray.

Millions of people simply chose to act like the pandemic was not happening: the deaths were inflated by doctors; the deaths were concentrated in the elderly and minorities, whose lives (implicitly) counted for less; masks were actually bad for you; there was a plot by prominent liberals to promote vaccines, or (depending on the mood) to delay them; the goal was to destroy the president, and to overthrow civil liberties. The president himself got COVID, received a monoclonal antibody before anyone could access that therapy, and then told his supporters that the disease was no big deal.

A tidal wave of misinformation, mixed with populism, threatened to consume the country in a bonfire of ignorance. The president, for his part, refused to commit to a peaceful transfer of power if he lost the election. In spreading lies about the integrity of the election, he found millions of ordinary people—and dozens of congressmen—willing to serve as his parrots. Not everyone who voted for Trump was a fool, and not all Trump voters were incapable of thinking independently. But the atmosphere of a personality cult was unmistakable, and it allowed millions of otherwise sane people to say and support crazy things.

Amongst his most ardent supporters, this was mass indoctrination, a phenomenon that many Americans had read about in other countries, but never expected to see in our own.

I was reminded of an essay by the conservative writer Thomas Sowell, who described the German descent into madness before World War II:

> The racial fanaticism of Hitler and the Nazi movement, which spread to the German generation of their day and led ultimately to the Holocaust, were not historically distinct characteristics of Germans as a people. On the contrary, the rise of such a man as the leader of such a people should serve as a permanent warning to all people everywhere who are charmed by charisma or aroused by rhetoric.

It occurred to me that my ancestors had faced the Depression and world wars, and they had done so soberly. They seemed to me to be made of stronger stuff than my contemporaries. The most repugnant aspect of the Trump years was not the president's behavior, but the moods and rhetoric of those who fell under his sway, especially those who knew better and made excuses for him.

But all along, I believed that in America there was a decent majority that craved a successful response to the pandemic. Such a majority cannot emerge when the only message is failure. From the earliest days, Americans had heard denial and resentment from their leaders. What would happen if someone gave them a vision of success? Optimism is an analgesic. Hope is a great salve. In a democracy, a leader should cling to these as to a life raft.

Success in controlling the pandemic is what I continued to urge at our weekly City and County meetings, though I noticed that the mayor was again being pulled in contrary directions. I felt relief that Libby Char would assume command of the Department of Health, but the mayor had little confidence in that institution in the short term. At a minimum, Libby would need months to make progress. The mayor's term of office would soon be coming to an end, and he didn't want it to finish with a prolonged shutdown.

In mid-September, a contentious argument erupted over the city's reopening plan. The mayor, assisted ably by Hiro Toiya, wanted a tiered system that specified what activity was allowed, and what wasn't, for different levels of transmission. Having been through the chaos of numerous city and state edicts, many of which were tied only loosely to epidemiology, this was an improvement. The problem, though, was that we had no scientific way of defining the boundaries of any given tier, nor could we say with precision which activities were safe in the gray zones of moderate transmission.

I argued, after conversations with Tim Brown and DeWolfe Miller, that the city should give Libby Char a week or two in her new position before committing to a reopening plan. We wanted to know the DOH's capacity to control a surge in cases before agreeing to an opening scheme. This floated like a lead balloon, and I was soon acutely aware of the limitations of being an "adviser" during a crisis. Instead, conversation turned to what should be allowed, and what shouldn't, with restaurants as a particular sticking point.

I found the prospect of returning to an *izakaya* for a glass of *sake* unappealing. There were data that indoor dining was a risk factor for contracting COVID, and that towns that restricted dining enjoyed lower overall disease burden. There were additional data that uncontrolled transmission would kill the economy, so I didn't see any upside to high-risk activities when case counts were high. I wanted to see an expansion of outdoor and takeout dining, with fairly radical relaxation of the rules governing pedestrian traffic in streets and even rooftops. But I thought it wise not to resume indoor dining until the case counts were at least low enough to qualify for the moderate tier.

Once again, though, I lost the argument, and it became evident that the mayor felt strong pressure to allow a broader range of economic activity, even if transmission remained widespread. Caldwell acknowledged the disagreement with his doctors during his announcement, which took away some of the sting. I found myself reflecting again on the nature of the relationship between leaders and advisers. No one had voted for me. I had no actual authority or responsibility for the city's plan. I could sulk and make myself a nuisance, or I could try to understand his competing priorities. That seemed a more productive path, and after making my points concisely, I let go of indoor dining.

What made the city's reopening more complicated was the state's determination to forge ahead with a tourism reopening. I supported welcoming travelers, and the purpose of the letter in June was to align the medical community with the economic interest in a way that didn't pit one against the other. But there were months of additional experience to guide us, and the results from islands that adopted flimsy testing protocols were not reassuring.

The limitation of one-test schemes was based on the natural history of the infection. There's a latency period between the time of infection and viral shedding. Though the time course has not been nailed down precisely, and there is likely a distribution across the population, I suspect this period averages three or four days. People then begin to shed virus, and symptoms (if they develop) occur shortly afterwards. Most people shed viable virus for seven to ten days, but they may shed RNA fragments for weeks. This creates problems in using tests (especially the more sensitive NAAT tests) for screening asymptomatic people. I can have a false negative if I test too soon, because the patient isn't yet shedding. Even if the latency period is only a day, a false negative can result from testing before exposure, as can happen prior to travel, or from an improperly collected test. On the other hand, I can have a false positive if I test too late, because I may be detecting nonviable virus in a patient already recovering from infection.

A good border control scheme would enforce a fourteen-day quarantine for people who don't want to test and require at least two time points in testing for everyone else. The state plan did neither of those things. Quarantine enforcement was still spotty, and there was no plan for post-arrival testing.

There was also a matter of priorities. Because transmission risk was associated with gathering, each community had to define the most crucial activities. The state hadn't yet reopened schools to in-class learning for a majority of Hawai'i's students. Even after vaccines became available, and the state prioritized teachers in its program, there were marked delays in resuming in-person education. The Kauaʻi group focused on this, and I joined an op-ed organized by Kapono Chong-Hanssen that encouraged Kauaʻi to take advantage of its superior disease control by getting more kids back into class. But the statewide picture was less positive, and after private meetings between the teachers' union and the Department of Education, it became clear that many kids wouldn't return to class until the summer of 2021. I thought this wasn't nearly good enough, and it represented a key failure of the state to prioritize the interests of children. This would have consequences that were negative to both the public health and economy. But kids didn't whine to politicians, nor did they decide who would be the next governor.

I shared my thoughts with reporters writing about the tourism plan and with my community online. I was a guest for Mel Rapoza and Charlie Iona, who had a nightly pandemic show on Facebook that was popular throughout the state. I also urged the new DOH leadership to push for stronger border protections.

I had no relationship with Lt. Gov. Josh Green. I thought his service early in the pandemic was useful, and in March I was grateful there was a doctor in the state government who was willing to question the narrative minimizing the threat. The second letter of our hui, establishing the concept of test-based border control, was successful because of its symmetry with his internal efforts. We wanted to leave the state room to improve its approach. The success of the Safe Travels plan, even if we arrived there through a circuitous route, would be the best outcome. But to succeed in epidemic control we needed to prevent the virus from crossing the border. That would require a more comprehensive plan for both testing and quarantine.

Not all was grim in the government as summer turned to fall. Libby Char moved quickly to reorganize the leadership at the DOH. The change in tone was immediate and positive. For the first time in months, I found myself in regular and friendly conversation with DOH officers. It was apparent that within that institution there was a great desire to succeed.

Given room to improvise, people there were eager to wrestle the virus. The DOH hotel quarantine program was Libby's first big win. Working through Eddie Mersereau, between mid-August and early October the department's capacity for quarantine grew from eighty to four hundred hotel rooms. Wait times on rooms also decreased, allowing the state to get people out of crowded houses before they infected their relatives. Eddie became a regular in the mayor's meetings, and this allowed a greater fusion of city and state efforts. Mayor Caldwell lavished resources in supporting him. This success was gratifying to me, as hotel quarantine had been my first drumbeat back in March and April.

The tier system, combined with universal mask use and a renewed focus on test-trace-isolate, paid dividends for O'ahu. Although transmission remained unsettlingly high during the fall and winter, it never exploded to the levels seen in August. Case counts, in fact, dropped gradually over a period of several weeks, allowing the island to advance tiers and open more activities. This was despite an influx of travel-related cases, as well as clusters that occurred in the restaurants. The success allowed Kirk Caldwell to hand his successor a pandemic infrastructure that worked.

The district health officers (DHO) on the Neighbor Islands assumed a more prominent role under Char's leadership. I began to understand that much of the trouble I had witnessed in the DOH was an O'ahu problem. Relations between the Health Department and the counties were much more congenial on the Big Island, Maui, and Kaua'i. During the bad days, in fact, the district health officers had got into the habit of piloting their own ships to protect each island. This partly explained the discrepant results between O'ahu and the Neighbor Islands. Janet Bereman, the DHO on Kaua'i, had a particularly strong record, and she soon became an important figure in the reorganized DOH leadership.

On September 10, introduced by JoAnn Yukimura, David and I met with Harry Kim, the Big Island mayor. Eric Honda, the capable DHO on the Big Island, attended the meeting. At this point, the Big Island was suffering through an uptick in cases, and unlike O'ahu, the island lacked the ICU capacity to absorb the blow. The Yukio Okutsu Veterans Home in Hilo experienced a particularly devastating outbreak that eventually killed dozens of residents. One of the deaths was the Reverend Richard Uejo, one of the state's last surviving WWII veterans. Kim was incensed. He nearly teared up speaking about the veterans. It was obvious he was determined to make changes at the facility. Soon afterwards he convinced Governor Ige to fire Avalon Health Care, the administrator.

Kim was thin and wiry, with a friendly smile that could turn to irritability in a heartbeat. In welcoming me, he showed graciousness. But as the subject turned to Yukio, I could sense his ferocious side. After summarizing his frustration with a few choice words, he stalked off, leaving his team to wrap up the meeting. I liked what I saw, and later I sent him a friendly follow-up message. But I wasn't sure how I could help him best.

The situation clarified in the coming weeks. I began to see COVID cases in Waimea, and it was obvious that there was community transmission on the Kona side of the island, as well as in a couple nursing facilities. I could identify at least two clusters, one within the Pacific Islander community in Kona, which continued to host large communal gatherings, and the other in the care homes. These were separate struggles, and each required a different containment effort. I began speaking regularly with Darragh O'Carroll, a bright ER doc who had taken over the testing operations for Premier Medical Group. Premier was Scott Miscovich's outfit, and Scott had built it into such a powerhouse that he was managing testing for COVID-free bubbles on the Mainland. O'Carroll was at this time the man on the spot in Hawaiʻi. The Premier guys had a piratical quality in the way they functioned. They were expert in the testing technology, but also willing to deploy it in unconventional ways. O'Carroll was working in contract with an anonymous benefactor from the tech industry who wished to improve testing on the Big Island. The combination of medical expertise, tech brains, and big capital was a potent one. The county merged their disease control effort with these companies, and the result was that Harry Kim had tools that few rural mayors in America could deploy.

In follow-up conversations, Kim coordinated outreach to the Pacific Islanders, and his team deployed testing to both nursing homes and crowded housing. This became part of an overarching infrastructure for testing. The county had access in Hilo to a NAAT machine, and they made plans to expand testing capacity. Premier acquired rapid tests for the mobile clinics, adding a more flexible dimension to the testing.

Kim also insisted on a modification of the Safe Travels plan for the Big Island. Working through Premier, he established post-arrival testing at the island's airports. The tests applied to people coming from the Mainland who had already taken a pretravel test. I wasn't convinced this would add much value, because it was too soon after the pretravel test. Ultimately the arrival testing did not catch a high rate of infections, but it caught a few. After traveling myself, I better appreciated the value of the extra test. Upon landing in Hilo, I had to go through an Army checkpoint manned by polite but well-armed guardsmen. Interisland travelers like myself were required to have a pretravel test from the neighbor island. But transpacific travelers, including those who had layovers on the Neighbor Islands, had to produce a pretravel test and then submit a post-arrival sample. The mere knowledge that this experience awaited me had served as a sobering reminder of the seriousness of the county in keeping disease out. Many people chose not to travel at all, or to take all necessary precautions to avoid a quarantine order at the airport.

As these plans unfolded, I looked at Harry Kim with increasing admiration. He was in his last months as mayor of the Big Island. He had not succeeded in his quest for a final term. But this disappointment also set him free. He cared not at all what others thought of him. He was the first mayor to insist on post-arrival testing for travelers, and this made him the first leader in Hawaiʻi to deploy rapid antigen tests at scale. Though the screening testing occurred only at the airport, it sparked a broader debate over the state's testing and border control scheme. This was an argument soon to spread to every county, with Kauaʻi in particular taking the lead. Kim also showed creativity in fusing the work of the district health officer with independent physicians and with industry. His was a multilayered system, and though no layer was a perfect defense, the net impact was to improve the security of the island.

The county smothered the fires in Kona and Hilo, and it reinforced its air border. Cases on the Big Island soon dropped. What looked like a wave of infection ended up being a splash. In Waimea, I saw fewer cases, and no one at Queen's North Hawaiʻi died. I enjoyed my new home and time with my family. The wide open beauty of Mauna Kea, snowcapped in the winter, with slopes dropping from towering heights all the way to my cottage, felt like the antidote to years of strain in the city. Layla found an Australian shepherd dog, and we strolled with him through acres of misty pasture, the blue sea off Hāmākua shining through trees and across our neighbor's fields.

An island defended is an island cherished. Harry Kim's style was at times eccentric, but his legacy in Hawai'i's greatest emergency is one that any leader would do well to imitate.

Chapter Thirteen

DELIVERANCE

DECEMBER 31, 2020

21,392
HAWAIʻI

18,648,989	79,231,893
UNITED STATES	WORLD

COVID-19 cases (data sources: World Health Organization and Hawaii Department of Health)

The day of the vaccine was like dressing up to go downtown. I wore my nicest shirt, and I made sure the nurses took a photo. I was never so excited to get a vaccine. As I entered the clinic, I realized I was participating in one of the great rituals of medicine. Vaccination is the archetype for progress in infectious diseases. Its history predates modern medicine, coming to the profession downstream from variolation, a technique by which practitioners in China protected their patients from smallpox by inoculating a sample of infectious material. The method traveled the Silk Road and became common practice for the Ottomans. It entered Africa before it arrived in Europe. A slave in early America described it to Cotton Mather, who was shocked by it and then promoted it in Boston. It was a gruesome curiosity when British physicians first described it at the Royal Society. To use the disease against itself! To coax the body, through the mysteries of immunity, to defeat the infection without recourse to drugs. The British had to overcome their horror at the thought of such a procedure, handed down to them from the ancient world. They did, and by developing art into science, they unlocked a revolution.

The COVID vaccines caused me anxiety, even though I was fully in alignment with the effort. No vaccines had ever been produced with anything like this speed. Within days of sequencing the virus, Pfizer and Moderna were developing messenger RNA vaccines. They compressed the phase three trials into just two months of follow-up, allowing the companies to thrash development time records. Previously the fastest vaccine production time was for the mumps, but that vaccine was created in the 1960s. Sequencing of SARS-CoV-2 to FDA emergency approval of the vaccine occurred in just eleven months.

Serious objections were, of course, raised to such a process. Was there sufficient transparency in the phase three trial data? Was two months of safety information enough to capture all the relevant side effects? Were pharmaceutical companies trustworthy partners for the government-financed effort? As with every other aspect of the pandemic, legitimate questions mixed with psychedelic conspiracies, making reasoned conversation difficult.

I thought there were fair reasons to worry about safety, and in particular I wanted more than two months of safety data. Coronavirus vaccines in domesticated animals had a mixed track record. Waning immunity and incomplete protection were issues. In some instances, antibodies induced by vaccination actually enhanced natural infection. There was no evidence of this in the phase three data, but how could the FDA be certain with such a limited observation window?

Time was a luxury the country lacked. During November and December, cases again surged. Hawaiʻi, as before, lagged a month or so behind. On the Mainland, deaths surpassed three thousand per day. This was equivalent to a 9/11 every twenty-four hours, week after week. To wait six months in such a context would have been ludicrous and cruel.

In North Hawaiʻi, I offered to go after the nurses and more frontline doctors. To my surprise, the administration asked me to go with the first wave. People were nervous. They wanted to see the infectious diseases doctor roll up his sleeve. I understood I had a second role to play here.

I wasn't just present to help people make sense of the disease, or to help treat it. I had a more soldierly task, to be first, and to suffer first if necessary. I did not resent this. It's a fine thing to be part of a profession that applies its principles first to its own leadership. And while I was anxious about the speed of the clinical trials, I thought the science was good.

It was in this feeling of optimism, seasoned with nervousness, that I presented my arm to the needle.

The vaccinations began in mid-December, but they were two-shot engagements, and I understood it would be months before the state could vaccinate enough people to knock the epidemic down. Although the development of the mRNA vaccines was a scientific triumph, production, distribution, and administration remained difficult. The federal government had prepared for this, purchasing supplies in advance of the clinical trials, in order to eliminate the usual delay between FDA approval and arrival of vaccine in clinics. This was the right move, as the likelihood that at least one vaccine would work was high. In the end, their efficacy surpassed all expectations. But the purchase was only one part of the chain, and the federal government struggled with the rest of it. The feds left distribution to states, which quickly bogged down in their efforts to get shots into arms.

The country had several hard months in front of it. These would be the deadliest months, as the third wave of the coronavirus surpassed all others in size and lethality. Back in May and June, when our hui first began planning in earnest for a reopening of tourism, the Mainland experienced twenty to thirty thousand cases per day. The debate then was whether that was too much to safely open the industry, and what safeguards would be appropriate. But by December, with the tourism economy tentatively open, the Mainland routinely reported more than two hundred thousand cases per day. California, a major source of visitors for the Islands, experienced such a rise in cases that the hospitals around Los Angeles began rationing care. Once again, the country was back in Italy, with the logarithmic growth of the virus straining even the

VARIANT DESIGNATION	COMMON NAME	NOTABLE MUTATIONS	CHARACTERISTICS
B.1.1.7	Alpha (UK)	**N501Y**, Δ69/70, others	50% increased transmission, increased severity
P.1	Gamma (Brazil)	**N501Y**, **E484K**, others	Reduced neutralization of convalescent and postvaccination sera
B.1.351	Beta (South Africa)	**N501Y**, **E484K**, others	50% increased transmission, reduced neutralization of convalescent and postvaccination sera
B.1.429	Epsilon (California)	**L452R**, others	20% increased transmission, reduced neutralization of convalescent and postvaccination sera
B.1.617.2	Delta (India)	**L452R**, others	50% increased transmission, increased severity

Figure 13.1 Data by Centers for Disease Control (CDC), table by the author. Reduced neutralization of convalescent and postvaccination sera refers to the variant's ability to evade immunity (either natural infection or postvaccination).

best attempts to scale up the human response.

In addition, there were descriptions of new coronavirus variants that appeared to be more transmissible and more lethal. The first well-described variant arose in the United Kingdom, but there were others in South Africa, Brazil, India, and even California. The United States did not routinely genotype coronavirus isolates, so the country was ignorant of circulating strains and their characteristics. The potential for vaccine escape—in which a circulating variant "escapes" the immunity generated by vaccines or natural infection—was my principal worry.

I thought the situation since the summer had changed. Not only was there a lot more disease, and potentially treatment-resistant disease, but the state was a few months away from protecting the population with a safe vaccine. The CDC issued a blanket recommendation during the holidays for people to avoid unnecessary travel. Catering to tourists in this context was ridiculous. I disagreed with politicians, increasingly eager to please the business community, who argued that Hawai'i should "live with the virus." I didn't want to live with it. I wanted to beat it, and the state finally had a tool that would allow it to accomplish that aim, provided it didn't sabotage its own effort. Who would be the last people to die of COVID before the vaccines were distributed? Who would suffer on the altar of an economic model that made no sense during a pandemic?

The actual risk from visitors was difficult to gauge. I repeatedly saw cases in the hospital of returning residents who had negative pretravel tests, then became sick after arrival. As expected, a single test wasn't perfect. But how imperfect was it? That was hard to measure precisely. A separate question was where to focus the limited post-arrival testing resources. It was notable that most of the travel-related cases I saw, both in the spring and winter, were returning residents, not tourists. It seemed plausible that Hawai'i's own residents were higher transmission risks than tourists, who had less contact with the local population. The state also had critical infrastructure workers who often were exempt from testing.

The lack of cases labeled "tourism" by the DOH wasn't entirely reassuring. Returning residents completed a pretravel test less often than

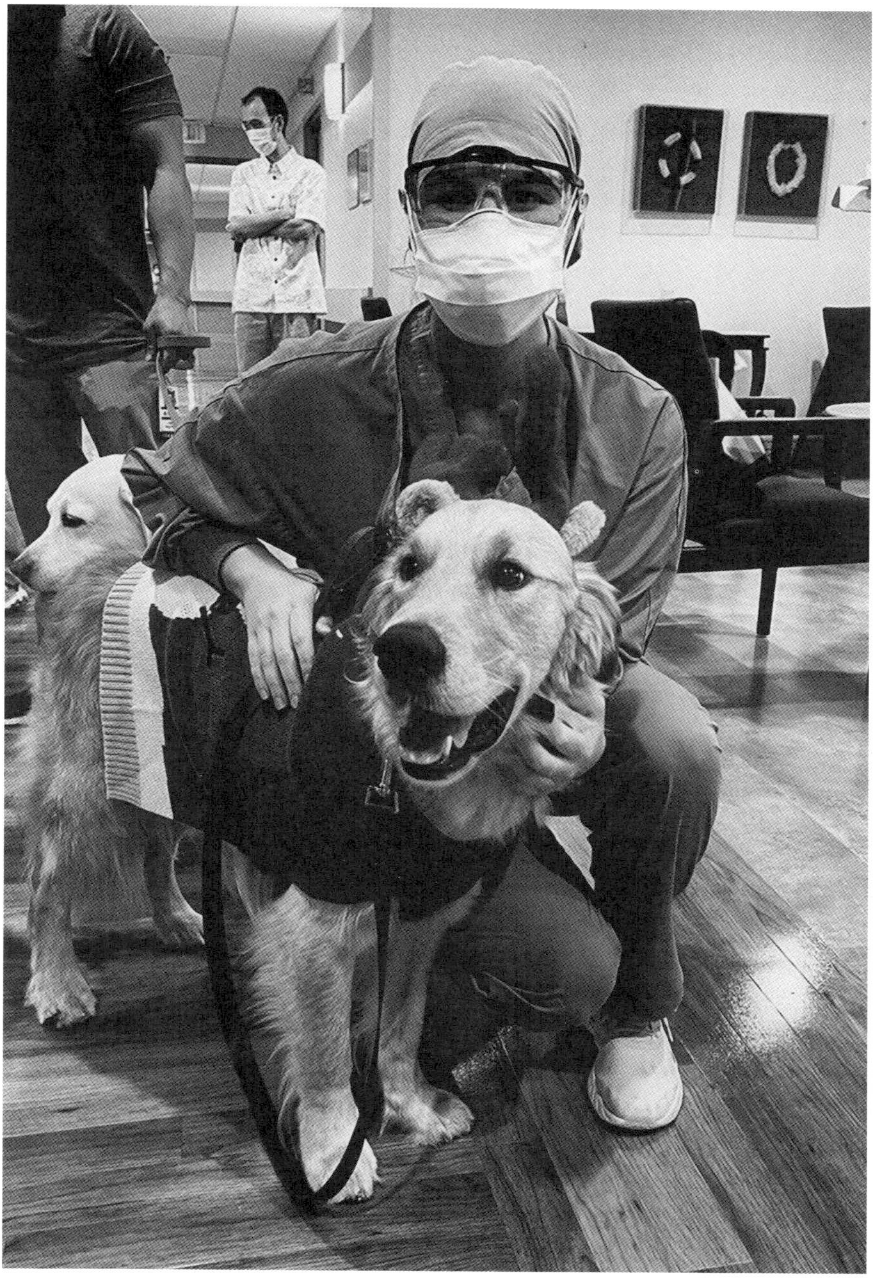

Nurse Kathleen Chamberlain pauses for a moment with a service dog on the COVID-19 unit. The hospital used dogs to help workers relieve stress.

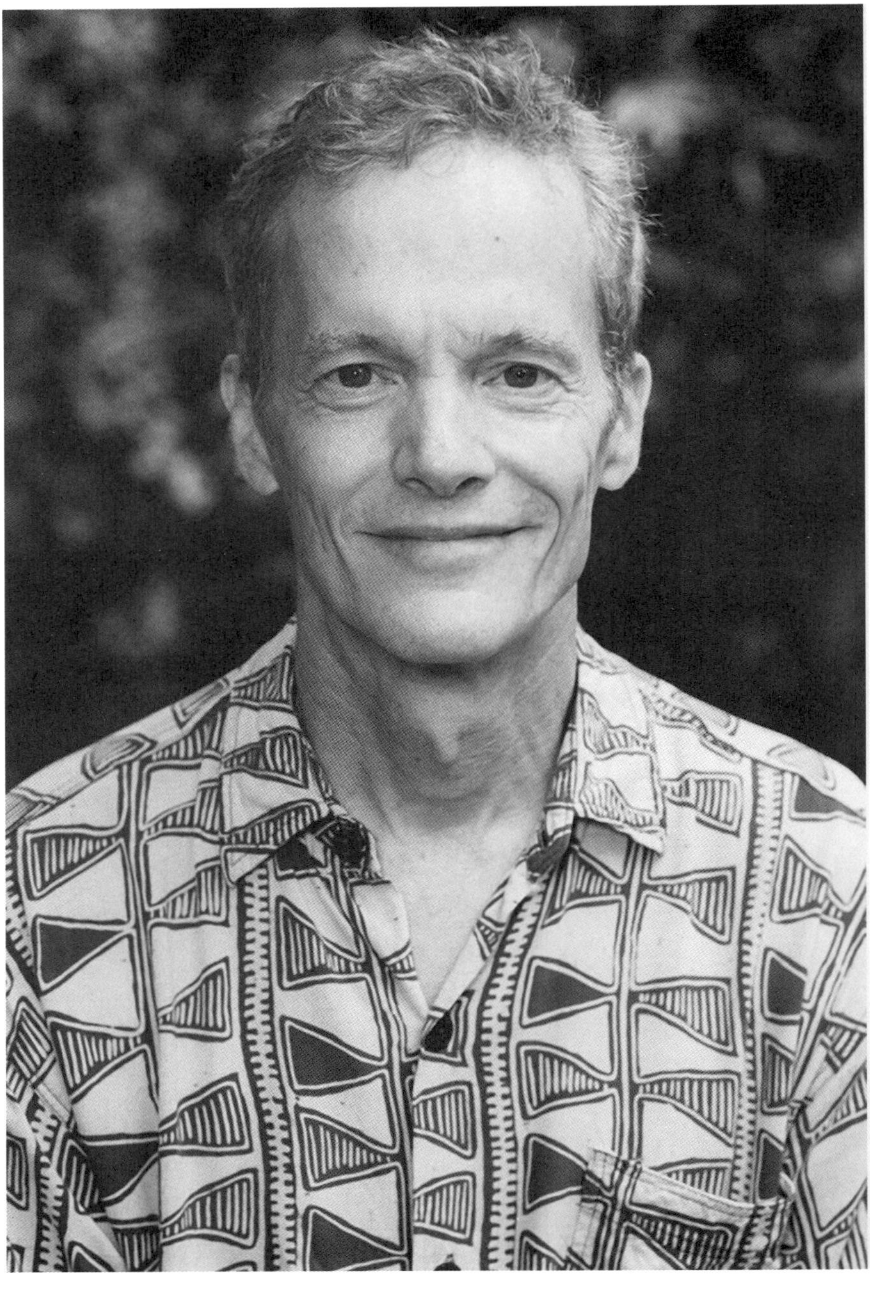

David Derauf, director of Kōkua Kalihi Valley, played a critical role in convincing the City and County and state governments to respond aggressively to the pandemic.

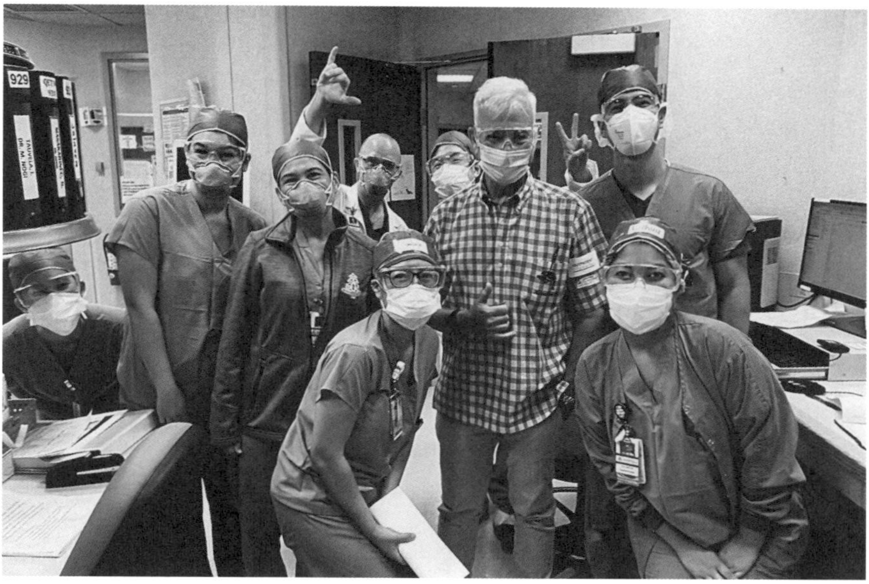

The mayor's visit wasn't reported but was well received by nurses and internists on the COVID unit.

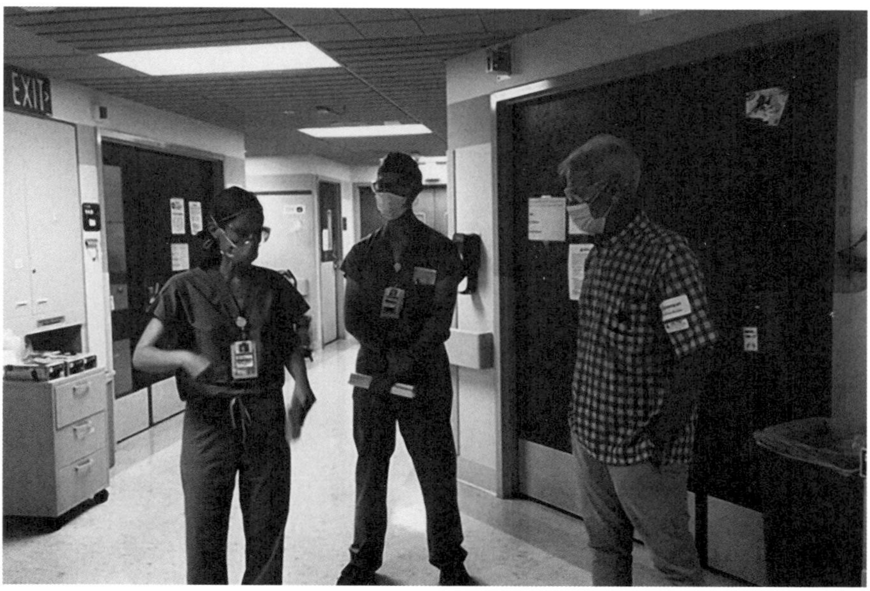

Honolulu mayor Kirk Caldwell (right) speaking with COVID internists Ryan Honda (center) and Malia Ramirez .

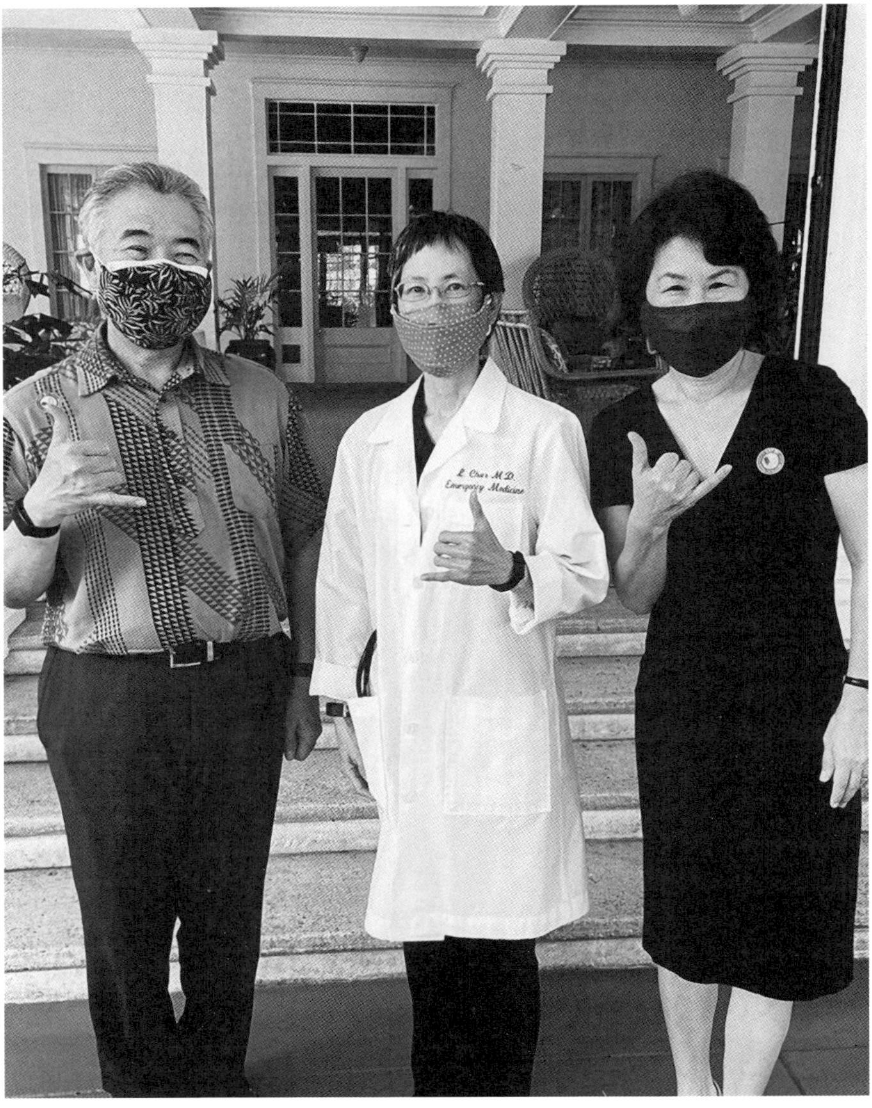

Libby Char (center), newly installed as director of health, enjoyed a light moment after vaccinating Governor David Ige and First Lady Dawn Ige.

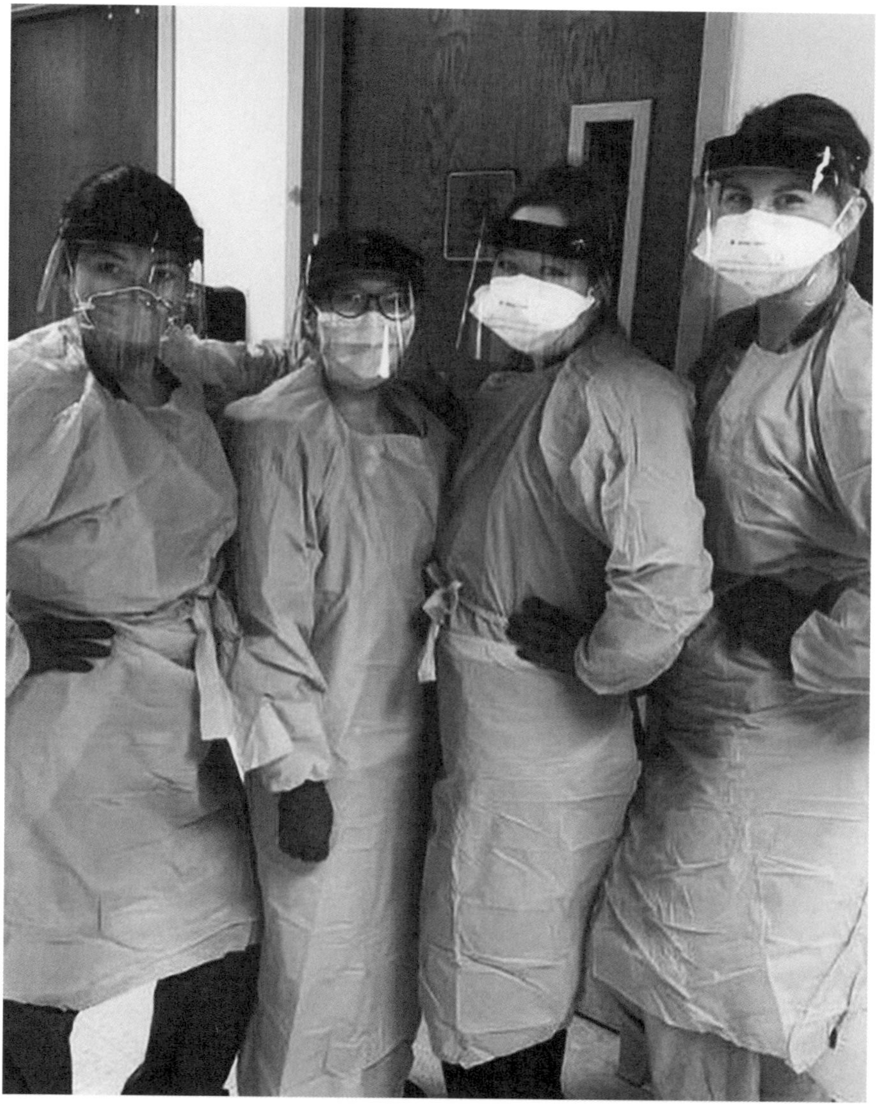

Left to right: Nurses Kuulehua Lorenzo, Candace Silva, Charlene Tanabe-Pang, and Kathleen Chamberlain work a shift on the COVID-19 unit at Queen's Tower 9 Diamond Head.

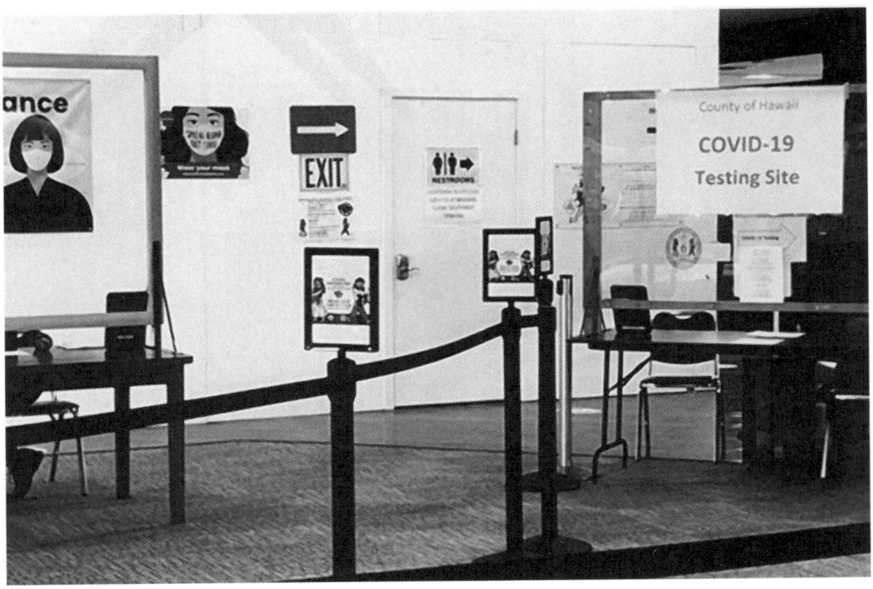

A testing station at Hilo International Airport on the Big Island. Manned by Hawaii National Guard and testing personnel, the station could go from empty (between flights) to processing two hundred people in less than an hour after a flight's arrival.

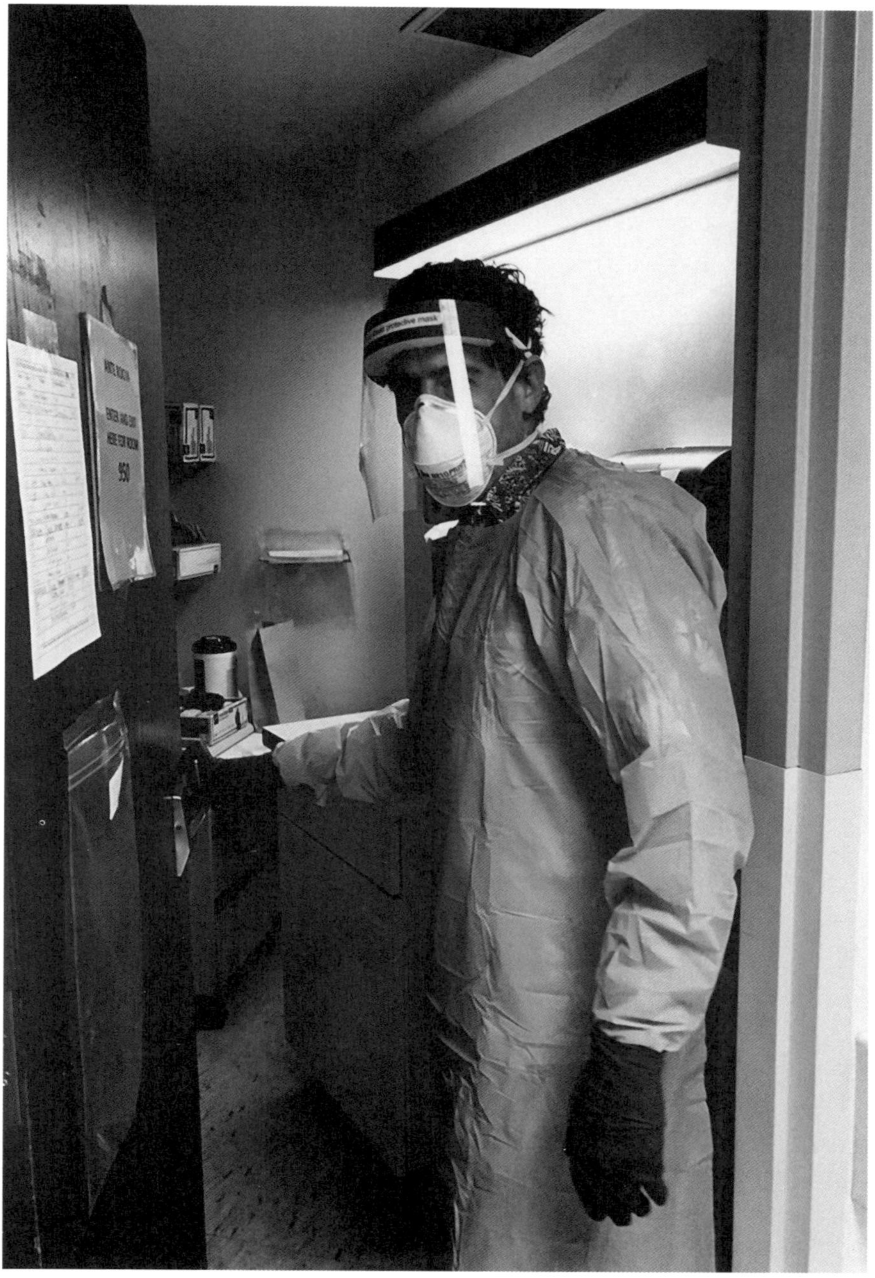

The author entering a COVID room with N95 mask, face shield, contact gown, and gloves.

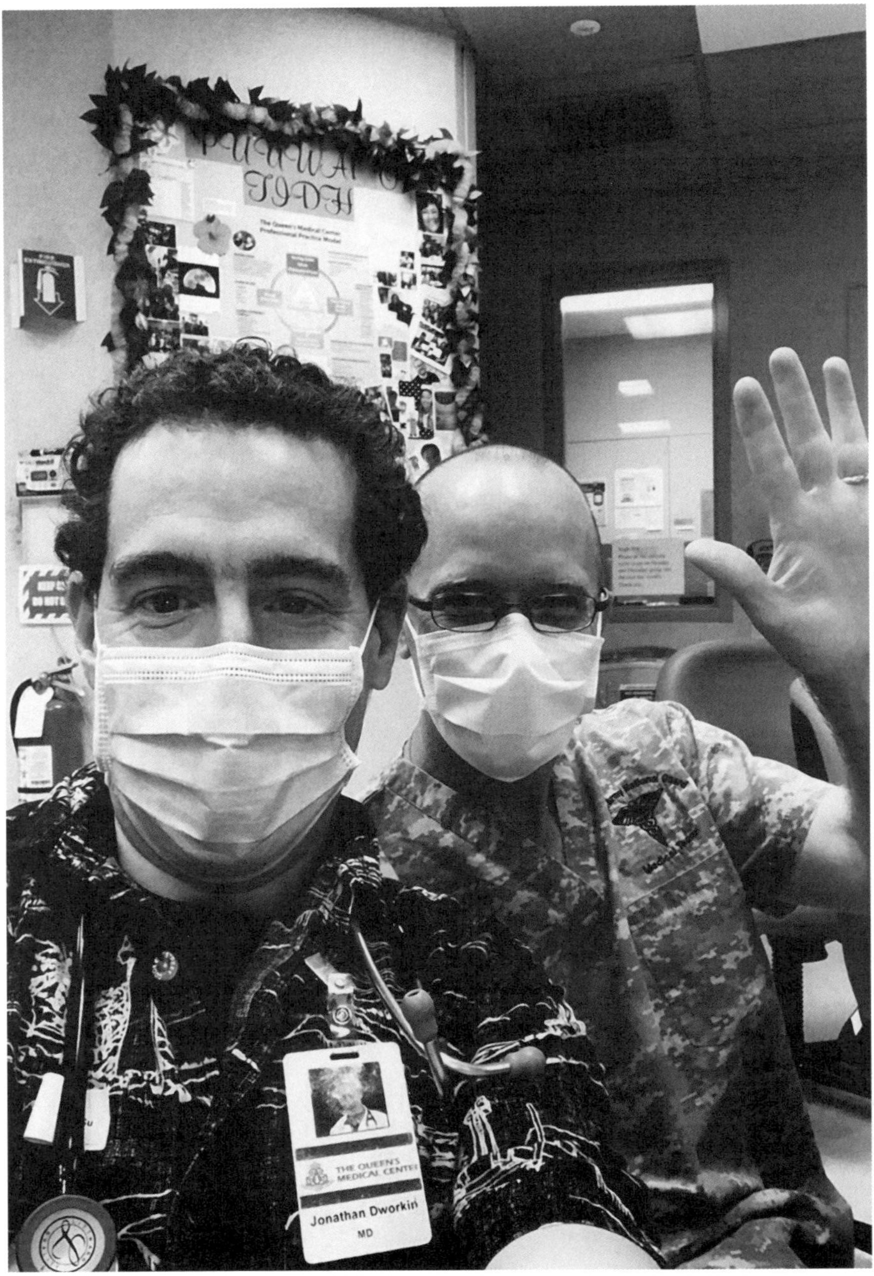

The author (left) with Lester Morehead at the nursing station, Tower 9 Diamond Head, July 2020.

tourists, choosing instead to "quarantine." But quarantine in Hawai'i was a paper tiger, with both the state and county governments admitting in private that they had no means of enforcing it at scale. I thought this was an error, and possibly the cardinal error, of the entire border control scheme. Without real quarantine, a traveler could evade any testing plan. These cases and their downstream infections were travel-related, even if they went undetected or had nothing to do with tourism.

It proved difficult to track down every case in the fall and winter, and to correctly determine travel links. The DOH had begun releasing cluster reports that attempted to identify the highest-risk activities, associated with the largest groupings of cases. Tourism rarely made it onto the cluster report. Church services, indoor dining, and work or home gatherings were the common culprits. But the DOH did detect a steady increase in travel-related cases after the tourism reopening in mid-October, and this played out differently on each island. On O'ahu, which had its own brisk epidemic, the travel cases remained a minority of the total. But on Kaua'i and Maui, which had mostly eliminated transmission, the travel reintroductions were a bigger problem. As cases steadily grew through October and November, the prospect loomed of the disease becoming endemic on both islands. Looking over at O'ahu, many people on Kaua'i felt it wise not to imitate that system.

We had some data from post-arrival testing to guide us. The Big Island did arrival tests on all Mainland travelers who had pretravel tests. This, of course, missed the people who did not test before flying (either because of an exemption or because of a plan to quarantine). That data, taken on people with a negative test within the past few days, showed a low incidence of disease amongst arrivals. The actual number was one in a thousand initially, and it climbed to two in a thousand as the Mainland epidemic worsened. As the test was done on arrival, not a few days after, it likely missed people in the latency period.

There was a small amount of data collected four days after arrival in a study conducted by DeWolfe Miller, and this showed a higher rate of infection. The number was six to nine times higher than the initial entry testing on the Big Island, with cases concentrated in returning residents. But the data was limited by selection problems, as only a tiny proportion of people invited to do a post-arrival test at four days showed up.

The district health officer on Maui, Lorrin Pang, did his own post-arrival testing. In order to get a higher rate of acceptance, he offered travelers a test at the time of departure, with the results kept confidential. This allowed him to accomplish two things. A much higher percentage of travelers agreed to be tested, and the average time between pretravel and post-travel tests was about a week. That was an ideal time interval. His data showed the incidence of infection was approximately seven per one thousand. That was a concerning number given the volume of travel through the state, though it, too, was limited by sample size.

Imperfect and conflicting data was the story throughout the pandemic. But it was obvious that the leakier the border, the higher the risk. I didn't need to know the precise rate of infection amongst travelers to understand the basic point, which was that the state was increasing the chance of a new wave of infection, possibly with a SARS-CoV-2 variant that would be more resistant to treatments or vaccines.

Mayor Derek Kawakami, again charting his own path, left the Safe Travels program in December, opting instead for a fourteen-day quarantine on all arrivals. In response, the epidemic on Kaua'i quickly plunged back towards zero. The Big Island remained in the program, but with Harry Kim's post-arrival testing as an additional safeguard.

Maui, on the other hand, kept to the basic Safe Travels program. Their experience was instructive. They saw a slow but steady rise in cases, and by January 2021, their epidemic on a per capita basis was similar to Mainland cities like Seattle and San Francisco. Gene sequencing data showed the majority of new cases were the variant first described in California. This was estimated by the CDC to be 20 percent more contagious, resistant to monoclonal antibody therapies, and possibly more resistant to vaccine-induced immunity. There's no way that variant got to Maui except by travel. In other words, Maui experienced exactly the scenario the Safe Travels critics feared.

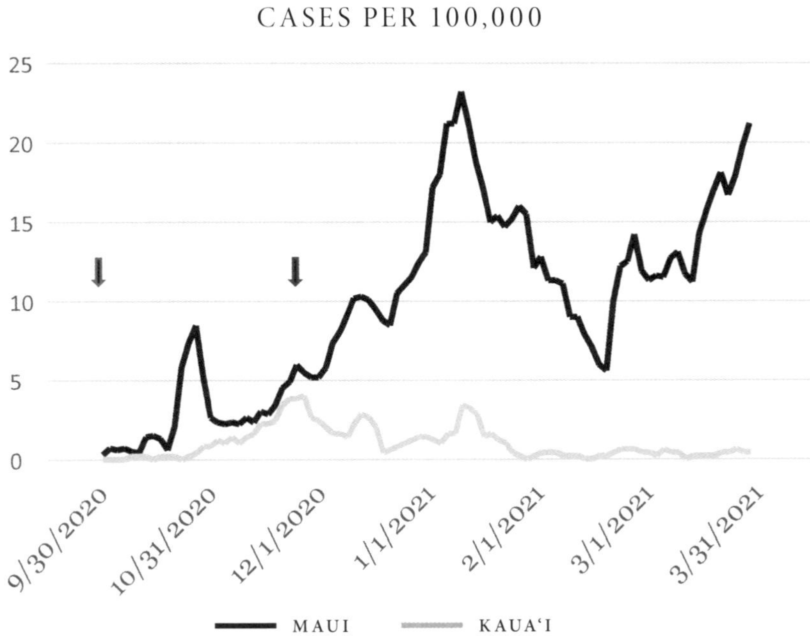

Figure 13.2 Data by the Hawaii Department of Health, graph by the author. First arrow indicates entry into Safe Travels on October 15. Second arrow indicates Kauaʻi's exit from the program and resumption of a mandatory, fourteen-day quarantine on December 1.

On Oʻahu, the effect of travel was less obvious, because the island started from a higher baseline of endemic disease. But the appearance of mutant SARS-CoV-2, in particular the California variant, indicated that the Safe Travels program was not preventing the importation of new and more resistant viruses. Edward Desmond, the director of the state lab, later provided a detailed breakdown of the variant problem in Hawaiʻi. By March 2021, variant strains accounted for a majority of cases statewide. On Oʻahu, the California variant was 59 percent of isolated cases. On Maui, that variant was 82 percent of isolated cases. The Big Island lagged behind, with a minority of cases identified as variants. Kauaʻi, being disease-free, had no data. As the variants became endemic on both Oʻahu and Maui—the two islands with the least border control—they threatened to seed additional outbreaks on the disease-free islands, and to undermine the enormous progress made by DOH workers and the state's vaccine program.

Cluster analysis done on Kaua'i, where Janet Bereman piloted a well-disciplined effort, also showed that the state was undercounting travel-related cases. The DOH typically reported cases in travelers and their immediate contacts as "travel" cases. But Bereman's work demonstrated that travel introductions extended out in concentric circles from the original infection, and that cases categorized as community-acquired could, in fact, have a travel origin. This is precisely what one would expect with a leaky border entry scheme.

DeWolfe Miller wrote a report, released November 30, 2020, on his post-arrival testing, and he did his best to interpret the data mess produced by the various testing schemes across the Islands. I have great respect for DeWolfe, and as I read his report, I was pleased to see us reaching many of the same conclusions. DeWolfe emphasized the multiplicative power of screening steps, in which the limited sensitivity of any one screen is offset by the benefit of sequential steps. In Safe Travels, this included the elements unrelated to testing, such as symptom checks. I agreed with him that testing resources, if limited, should be directed towards the highest-risk travelers, and that testing exemptions for travel should be reduced. DeWolfe was also open to post-arrival testing, though he wanted to see it targeted:

> Recommendation for a **second post-arrival** [emphasis added] test may be justified and more efficient if consideration is given to a more defined group of arrivals, specifically **returning residents** [emphasis added]. A rapid antigen capture test on arrival would be cost-efficient and implementable.

I preferred a quarantine and a second test around day five. But here was a reasonable compromise, if anyone would take it. Despite all the noise in the press, and the impassioned arguments between activists and government, the actual science suggested it was possible to allow travel, provided the state maintained the security of its border. But getting that right meant increasing, not decreasing, the existing protections.

The state's unwillingness to accommodate contrarian voices led to dissent within both the government and the community, dooming a unified plan. The Department of Health grew tired of chasing down test results that turned positive after visitors arrived in state. This led to a DOH rule change, announced in late November 2020, that required all pretravel testing results be available prior to boarding. Given the surge of cases on the Mainland, and delays in testing, this further impeded visitors.

Due to the action of the mayors, Hawaiʻi entered 2021 with a patchwork of county-specific travel requirements. All of this frustrated the tourism industry and discouraged people from coming to Hawaiʻi. There was an industry-driven effort in the state House, known as HB 1286, to impose a single, unified system based on the Safe Travels framework. But this died in the legislature, and though I had championed a unified approach early, I saw the death of a statewide plan as a good thing. Any universal plan should have improved the common safety, not undermined it. I also thought the governor and mayors should preserve their power to protect the border, as they were better positioned than legislators to respond to emergencies in real time.

Taking a step back from these controversies, it's fair to ask: Who travels—relying on questionable safety protocols—during a deadly respiratory pandemic? There are people who can't avoid travel because it's essential for their work. There's the critical infrastructure group, which includes the military and healthcare sectors. There are also people who have family needs and emergencies. But tourism is a different creature. No one "needs" a vacation at a five-star hotel. Air travel, despite the belated attempts by industry to enforce mask use, was intrinsically high-risk. Data reported in Canada (there was no reporting requirement in the United States) revealed that thousands of domestic and international flights arriving in that country during the fall and winter carried active infections. The number of infected flights in the United States during that same period was almost certainly much higher. And how could it be otherwise? The industry's hostility to using rapid antigen tests on all

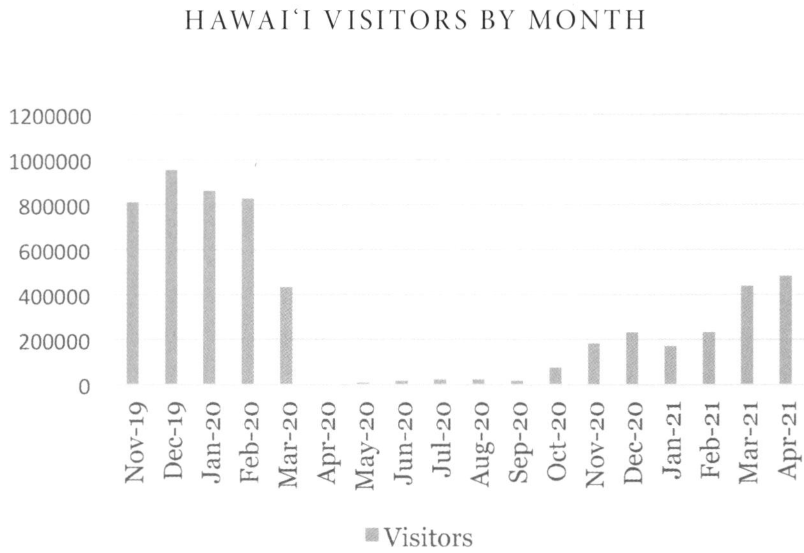

Figure 13.3 Data by Hawaii Tourism Authority, graph by the author.

passengers made it impossible to keep virus off the planes.

Even an airplane crew with meticulous attention to cleaning, paired with a modern ventilation system, couldn't escape the basic reality imposed by cramming hundreds of people into an enclosed space. And that's to say nothing of hours spent in airport security lines, in predeparture hangars, at baggage carousels, or time spent on the ground, some of it with ventilation systems off, during aircraft maintenance and ground transport.

Encouraging this activity without rigorous screening protocols struck me as the definition of "unintelligent." The CDC agreed, bluntly warning Americans not to travel during the winter months. Hawai'i's course was at odds with both the science and the federal recommendations.

Who, exactly, was Hawai'i attracting during these months of daily record deaths? And should the state have even tried to cater to such people?

These were inconvenient questions, and with billions of dollars at stake, no one in power wanted to ask them. But many people in Hawai'i noticed, and the state's already negative attitude towards tourism deteriorated further. A survey in December 2020 showed sentiment towards the tourism industry had reached its lowest point since the 1980s. The rebirth of the industry wouldn't begin in earnest until the spring.

The violent aftermath of the presidential election in Washington, DC, was a dispiriting event, but it shouldn't have surprised anyone. Those who had been paying attention to the president's rhetoric, a group that included many of his estranged former advisors, predicted months in advance his unwillingness to accept defeat. The people spreading pandemic disinformation intersected with those promoting election lies, as these conspiracies overlapped and traveled in the same social forums. But I was grateful that the violence was brief, unsuccessful, and universally condemned.

More pressing locally were the changes in county leadership. Kirk Caldwell and Harry Kim were no longer on the scene. On the Big Island, the new mayor, Mitch Roth, did not initially commit to maintaining Kim's approach, although he later extended the post-arrival testing program. His counterpart on O'ahu, Rick Blangiardi, had spoken of opening bars prior to taking his oath. With tourism remaining in deep freeze, there was a growing and understandable appetite to open the local economy.

My first interaction with Blangiardi came on January 7. I was not confident he would keep a medical advisory group, especially one handed off from his predecessor that would tell him things he didn't want to hear. To his credit, that's exactly what he wanted. A healthy argument erupted over the mayor's desire to dispense with Caldwell's tier system and get more businesses open. I pointed out that Caldwell had struggled most in the absence of a tier system, as he shouldered the blame for every decision impacting business. The whole point of his tiers was to depoliticize those decisions and lash them to the case counts. The new mayor could disregard that, but making those decisions by whim or fiat was unlikely to please anyone. I urged some kind of objective system, whether it be a tier or something new. In the end, he kept the tiers through March, which helped keep cases low in the period before the vaccine program ramped up.

The new mayor had coached youth sports, and rather than opening bars, I suggested he focus on kids and schools. What was the plan to vaccinate teachers? The benefits of prioritizing education were myriad. Most kids do better with in-person school, and the most unfortunate kids need it for nutrition and to escape domestic dysfunction at home. There's long-term social and economic benefit to getting children back into school, as well as short-term economic benefit to their parents. The new mayor wanted to open something, that was clear enough. I urged him to choose the right thing, and to be willing to fight for it.

Blangiardi's background in business also made him an ideal person to work with in revisiting some of the pandemic's earlier missed opportunities. Under its previous leadership, the DOH was not enthusiastic about developing testing locally. It had also not been open to private efforts to create app software to assist in coordination of test results, contact tracing, and quarantine services. These were key pieces of pandemic infrastructure that the state had not sufficiently developed. But they were also business opportunities for local entrepreneurs. With Libby Char now at the helm of the DOH, a pro-business mayor in Honolulu, and new stimulus coming to the county from the Biden administration, I pushed one final time to channel some resources into the city's nascent biotech industry. In an internal memo dated March 4, I addressed Mayor Blangiardi:

> One important difference between a competent response to the pandemic, which Hawaiʻi has already achieved, and a truly excellent one, will be the kind of infrastructure the City of Honolulu builds in order to prepare for future epidemics. When the virus hit last March, we had no capacity to test for the disease. This made the hospitals unsafe, and it left the entire city vulnerable. As a doctor, that's an experience I hope never to repeat.
>
> An attempt was made to build up local testing capacity during the emergency, and after weeks of hard work we were partly successful. But because we purchased testing systems designed out of state, we remained susceptible to supply chain disruptions, which hampered our efforts well into the summer.
>
> There exists within the city tremendous entrepreneurial talent. There's no reason why Honolulu cannot emerge from this pandemic with a small but

> well-regarded tech industry. Key areas of interest for pandemic response are biotechnology and software. Biotech is important because the city should have the capacity to produce its own rapid tests for any emerging pathogen. This is simpler than it used to be from a manufacturing standpoint, and tests can actually be made on island. Software and app development is another key resource, as it allows rapid notification of test results, contact tracing, and quarantine service coordination.
>
> Within the Health Department last year there was hostility to these ideas, and as a result not much was accomplished. However, with the leadership change on the state side, and new money coming in the form of federal stimulus, there's an opportunity to revisit these nondecisions.
>
> The beauty of building these industries locally is that it will provide a future mayor with useful tools to respond to problems in real time. It will also provide good jobs that attract talented people to the city and entice them to stay. "Shut it down" was always a clumsy strategy for combating the pandemic, and at best it was a tool of last resort to be used in an emergency. The truly dynamic places in the world relied on the ingenuity of their people and their businesses, partnering with government, to allow society to function through the pandemic.
>
> This seems to me a worthy priority for your administration, and one that could have positive and even historical consequences for Honolulu. Please give it your consideration, and take advantage of any opportunity that crisis presents you.

Having recently taken office, the mayor's administration was in its early phase, and he was working hard to establish a productive relationship with the state government. I'm not sure how much of an impact this letter had on his thinking, but he seemed open to it. I was pleased to be able to speak his language.

My involvement in the mayor's medical advisory committee came to an end the final week of March. With the vaccine program taking off in Honolulu, a new surge of cases prompted re-evaluation of the utility of the tier system. I thought it wise to stick with the tiers, and to continue to knock down transmission until the state vaccinated a majority of the local population. That was consistent with the recommendations coming from both the CDC and the DOH. But having waited to vaccinate most of the elderly, Blangiardi felt compelled to open things as quickly as possible. This included opening high-transmission venues like bars and weddings, which undermined the tier system. I disagreed, and I wanted to see far more vaccinated and the local epidemic in decline before we loosened public health restrictions. But I also understood that the tiers were never intended to last forever, and that vaccines were a far more promising strategy for disease control. The mayor had listened to us in January, when the vaccination program was just beginning, and in putting off his preferred approach, he had bought the city time to vaccinate tens of thousands of its most vulnerable residents.

The vaccines had transformed the situation since the fall, when Honolulu created the tier system. The risk in the spring of 2021 was an increasing incidence of variants that threatened the medium- to long-term success of the state's efforts. With Libby Char advising him from the DOH, I was confident that the mayor had access to bright and well-intentioned people in the medical community. The advisory committee, in my view, had outlived its usefulness. I felt it was time to get out of the way. I submitted a resignation letter, and after a brief and friendly chat with the mayor, my role advising the City of Honolulu came to an end.

The vaccination program began slowly, but in January it picked up steam. The day I received my second shot, the clinic was humming, with more than eighty vaccines administered. That was a sizable number for a town of ten thousand, and the hospital soon expanded to nearly two hundred shots per day. Now, instead of distribution and administration, supply again became the bottleneck. The state needed more vaccine, because the demand from the community surged. Shots in arms became the mantra. Could the state avoid a growth in cases long enough to get a few thousand more shots in arms? A few ten thousand? Each blip in the data was now measured against this background of vaccination and rising group immunity.

One interesting aspect of the early vaccine program was the sudden success of the American and UK efforts. The two countries were amongst the worst in the world at disease control and had some of the highest mortality rates. Anglo-Americans proved ill-suited for the drudgery of contact tracing and self-isolation, whereas Germans and Norwegians cooperated well with their government efforts. But the science was a different matter. Some of the best clinical trials during the pandemic were published in the UK. The American vaccines, using novel mRNA technology, were the best in the world and a triumph of American innovation. Both countries moved with alacrity and supercharged mass vaccination programs while their European counterparts foundered in red tape. By March, the UK was seeing sustained drops in case counts and deaths, while France and Germany began to suffer an additional wave. Amongst the British in particular there was a sense of schadenfreude as the country finally saw a concrete benefit emerge from its painful divorce from Europe.

The Israelis—another laggard in disease control—had the most successful vaccine program in the world, reaching a majority of their elderly population by February. Like the United States, they prioritized elderly and high-risk adults first. I followed their data daily, and I was relieved to see a drop in hospitalizations and cases amongst elderly Israelis. Later this extended to their other demographic groups, lining up nicely with the order of vaccination.

But there was also a lot of noise in the national data, with some countries (e.g., South Africa) recovering from case surges despite nonexistent vaccine programs, and others (e.g., Chile) experiencing new surges of cases despite early success in getting people vaccinated. Some countries had access to mRNA vaccines, which proved more effective against viral variants, while others relied on Chinese vaccines that were less successful. To make matters more confusing, the presence of more contagious variants in some countries increased the threshold needed to achieve herd immunity. It wasn't clear what number a country needed to hit with a given vaccine in order to send its epidemic into permanent decline. Based on the Israeli experience, in which an mRNA vaccine was used against the UK variant, I suspected it was 60–70 percent. The number was higher for the India variant, which was even more transmissable and began replacing the UK variant in the summer. Early on, there was also a lack of data about the duration of protection and the degree to which vaccination prevented asymptomatic transmission.

All of these concerns needed to be addressed, and they had enormous implications for what behavior should be allowed, and when. But these details would become clear over time. Data trickled in steadily in March

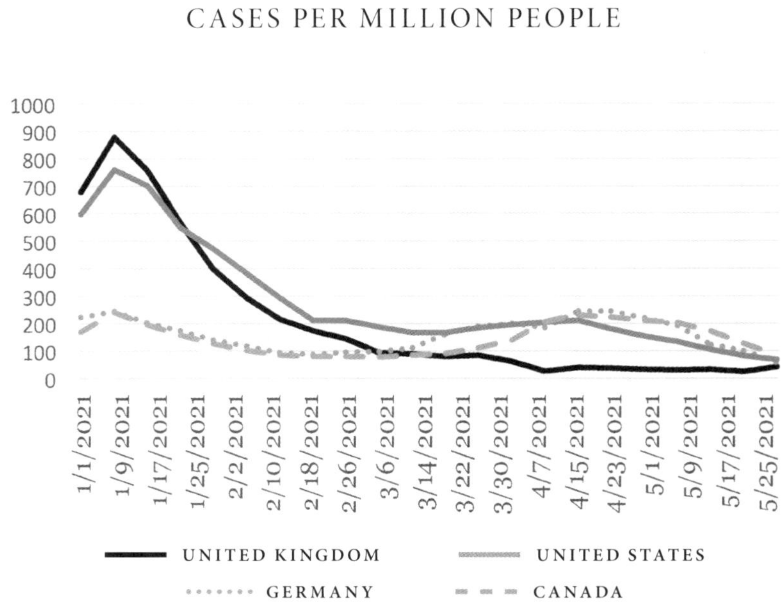

Figure 13.4—British success. Despite a worse epidemic, the rapid rollout of vaccines in early 2021 allowed the UK to outperform Germany and Canada, which suffered late waves during slow vaccination programs. Graph by the author. Data from Our World In Data.

and April, most of it affirming the value of the mRNA vaccines. I suspected we would not eliminate the disease. It had already found its way into animal reservoirs, and vaccine protection would not be complete. In countries with less access to mRNA vaccines, the death toll would remain high, and the United States would need to organize efforts to supply them with the new technology. But with a new president in the White House, and additional economic relief on the way, I was confident the United States would turn the corner. The violence in Washington, DC, had a subtle effect on people. America looked over the edge of the abyss, and didn't appreciate the view. The tolerance for fact-free commentary dropped. Instead, the Biden administration talked of one hundred million vaccine doses in one hundred days, a goal they handily exceeded.

In Hawaiʻi, doctors and nurses stood tall. Amongst the states, Hawaiʻi had the lowest rate of infection and death. Just as importantly, its citizens shared a common reality. The state exited the maelstrom unscathed by paranoia and demagogic visions. In the aftermath, the people beheld with renewed wonder the beauty and health of their islands. ☙

Chapter Fourteen

CONCLUSIONS

FEBRUARY 28, 2021

26,723
HAWAIʻI

28,174,978	113,472,187
UNITED STATES	WORLD

COVID-19 cases (data sources: World Health Organization and Hawaii Department of Health)

It's my hope that in reflecting on the experiences of Hawaiʻi during the pandemic, the reader is disabused of any notion that the state's response to the crisis was an unqualified success. It's easy to glance across the Pacific from the perspective of the US Mainland, observe the lower mortality rate in Hawaiʻi, and conclude "Ahh yes, it's good to be an island state." There's no doubt that geography and demography were critical factors in the success of Hawaiʻi. But if the only message that emerges is that of triumph, it will be a false narrative, and the story of the pandemic will resemble mythology more than history.

Even before considering what the state did well, it's prudent to challenge the assumption that the state did, in fact, do well. Compared to many jurisdictions on the mainland United States, Hawaiʻi's mortality rate was indeed low. But that's a simple bar to clear given the debacle that characterized the general American response. Compared to its peers in the Asia-Pacific region, Hawai'i looks decidedly mediocre. Judged by the death toll, the success of the state hovers in between that of its highly successful Asian neighbors and that of the country of which it's a part. This puts Hawai'i in the same range as the more successful Scandinavian countries like Denmark and Norway. Not bad, but not even in the same ballpark as places like New Zealand or Taiwan that made disease eradication their policy. Like those countries, Hawai'i had the advantage of sealing its border early, and its failure to replicate their success reflected a deep ambivalence on the part of its government to succeed in controlling the epidemic.

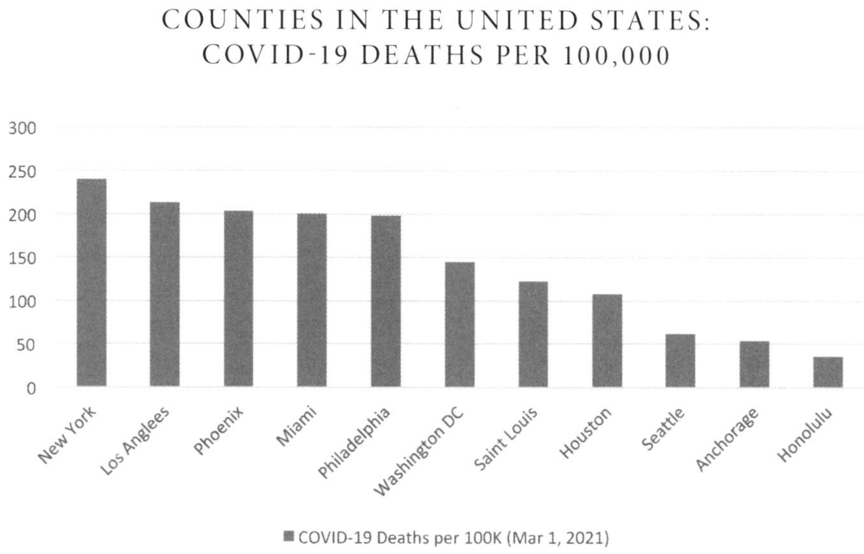

Figure 14.1 Data by US News (USA Facts). Graph by the author. Mortality data reflects the county in which each city sits.

Comparisons between countries are difficult. For some countries, like Russia and China, data may not be reliable if it collides with political narratives. For others, the lack of access to testing makes the data unreliable. The widespread availability of effective vaccines for wealthier countries (especially the US and UK) in March and April of 2021 makes comparisons in disease control beyond that time point less meaningful, as differences are increasingly driven by access to vaccines. Even in the UK and US, it's likely that SARS-CoV-2 cases will occur for years. But in countries with good vaccine programs, that will no longer correlate with full hospitals and large mortality events. Once the vaccines defang the epidemic, measuring case counts will be less meaningful.

With these caveats in mind, a close look at the data internationally through early 2021 shows three major patterns in the pandemic.

In the West, broadly defined as Europe and the Americas, there was uncontrolled disease spread and an associated mass mortality event, not brought under control until the implementation of effective mass vaccination programs.

In the developing world, a more complex pattern unfolded. In Africa, there was widespread disease, but not high mortality. The reasons for this are not yet entirely clear, but they likely relate to demographic and geographic variables in those countries. India followed a pattern similar to Africa initially, but it began to diverge in the spring of 2021 as variants spread rapidly across the country. This late wave, which was all the more tragic because it occurred after effective vaccines had become available in wealthier countries, caused the highest case and death counts in the world. Thousands of people died in India because hospitals ran out of beds, oxygen, and other critical supplies. This highlighted the failure to distribute vaccines quickly and equitably, a task that was important both to lower the mortality in poorer countries and to prevent them from becoming breeding grounds of virus variants that escape vaccine immunity. The disaster in India—and the threat it posed to the global containment effort—proved once again that there was no safety for anyone in allowing uncontrolled transmission.

In the Asia-Pacific region, there was excellent disease control and low mortality, which was threatened in early 2021 by delays in rolling out effective vaccine programs.

The painful contrast between Asia and the West prior to the availability of vaccines, which cannot be attributed to wealth disparity, reveals not just policy differences, but a divergence in the entire mindset of disease control. This is no mystery. The WHO's Mike Ryan identified the key dynamic as early as March 2020:

> Be fast. Have no regrets. You must be the first mover. The virus will always get you if you don't move quickly.... If you need to be right before you move, you will never win. Perfection is the enemy of the good when it comes to emergency management. Speed trumps perfection. And the problem in society we have at the moment is everyone is afraid of making a mistake, everyone is afraid of the consequence of error. But the greatest error is not to move. The greatest error is to be paralyzed by the fear of failure.

It's an inconvenient truth that at key moments during the state's pandemic response there was strong institutional pressure to do nothing at all. Like employees caught sleeping in their cubicles, some officials proved more expert at manufacturing excuses for inactivity than in articulating any plan to defeat the virus. This often took the form of fatalism over disease control, with talk of the "inevitability" of a respiratory virus spreading through the population. At other times turf was the excuse, and the authorities reminded those who wanted action to keep to their lane. When all else failed, the prophets of inertia would roll out the economy as their idol, insisting (without evidence) that any action to control the disease would stifle the free market and hurt the common people.

All of this, I hope the reader understands, is BS. It was painful for people to change the way they worked. It was hard to stand up new systems on short notice. It was awkward to insist to colleagues in parallel agencies that they needed to reimagine their roles—and in fact reimagine the role of government—in the context of a fast-moving emergency. It was much easier to smile knowingly and explain "how things work."

The unwillingness of Hawai'i's physicians to play along was, I realized with time, our superpower. I felt particularly blessed, because I had good colleagues, not the least of whom was David Derauf, who encouraged my contrarianism. We weren't alone, and we soon found doctors, nurses, public health experts, and activists organizing on each of the islands. The difference between success and failure relied on the emergence of leadership not from above, but from below.

To the extent that Hawai'i succeeded in demonstrating a competent public health system, it did so because of the persistent pressure by

COVID-19 DEATHS PER 100K (MARCH 19, 2021)

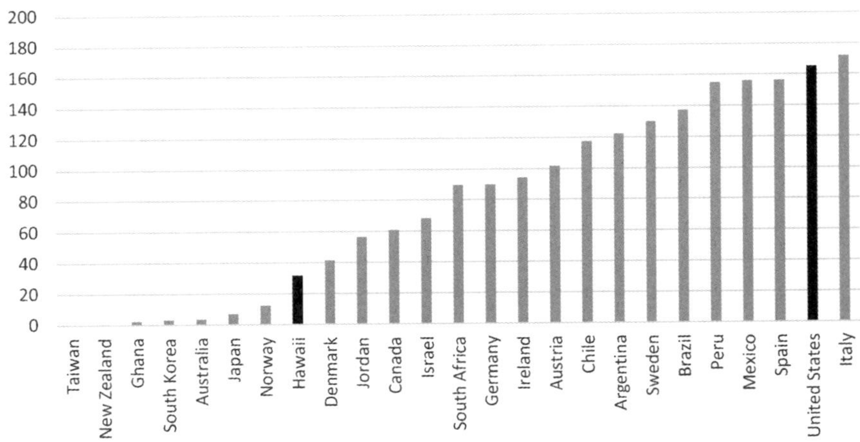

Figure 14.2 Data Source—Johns Hopkins University Coronavirus Resource Center. Graph by the author. Hawai'i separated from US total.

these individuals, and in the teeth of opposition from parts of the establishment. But once Hawai'i succeeded, the state quickly unlocked the talents of dozens of people in its health department, and of hundreds in other agencies and NGOs.

If there's a conclusion to draw here, it's that bureaucrats can't be counted on to provide leadership in moments of crisis. Bureaucrats are not leaders, even if they hold titles of authority. Politicians, for the most part, can't be counted on either, because they are enmeshed in electoral considerations. They often don't even interpret those correctly. I was perplexed by how frequently I heard politicians of both parties talk about living with the virus, as if a virus was another constituent they could accommodate, when I was sure the most popular thing was to beat it soundly, and reap the benefits.

Leadership is a nebulous concept, but in crisis it is everything. As much as I wished to avoid administrative tasks before the pandemic,

I learned that without sensible people shaping the conversation at the state's leading institutions, there was simply no chance of a successful outcome. Leadership matters. And Hawai'i needed doctors and nurses to show it. That they did so was not inevitable, and their ability to influence the trajectory of the disease in Hawai'i was the result of months of persistent, uphill struggle. Given the prospect of a mass mortality event looming over the state, they learned to not respect the lanes of power too much, and to intrude on the business of government with the urgency of knowledge and experience.

There was one jurisdiction in Hawai'i that committed to eradicating the virus. Kaua'i had no less dependence than any other island on tourist dollars, and like the rest, it was trapped in a larger and dysfunctional state and federal system. Kaua'i had the advantage, however, of an excellent district health officer and a mayor who worked well with her. Janet Bereman and Derek Kawakami stand apart from all other officials in the state as people who took the task of disease eradication with the utmost seriousness. They understood the vulnerability of their island, which lacked critical care beds, to a serious epidemic.

In the beginning, when Kawakami announced that the emergency was indefinite, he prepared his people for an extended disruption. Later, he resisted pressure from the state government and the media to cede control over his island's border to the authorities on O'ahu. He made no promise to be consistent with border policies either, insisting that he needed to respond to events in real time. In these comments he showed that he fundamentally understood the nature of the problem, and that others did not. In a boxing match you don't commit yourself to one style of defense in order to "be consistent." Consistency is no virtue in a boxing match. Not getting knocked out is the virtue. In resisting Honolulu, Kawakami never made a fuss, but he didn't back down either.

The argument over whether it was possible to eradicate a respiratory epidemic in Hawai'i was settled, in the affirmative, by its most under-resourced county. Kaua'i's case and mortality rate place that island within the category of highly successful Asia-Pacific states. As such, they enjoyed a more open society during the fall and winter—and less disruption to school and family life. Kauaʻi also had the fastest-paced vaccination effort in the state. In every healthcare category that mattered, they excelled. In achieving their aim of a disease-free island, they became an example of what the entire state could have achieved if the political will had existed to strengthen the public health infrastructure early in the pandemic and to maintain stronger control of the border.

A common retort is to point to Kauaʻi's small size, less than one hundred thousand people, and argue that such a plan would never have been possible in the larger counties. It's true that the short-term economic pain experienced on Kauaʻi was steeper than in the other counties, particularly when it was the sole island to maintain a strict, fourteen-day quarantine. But the criticism of Kauaʻi ignores the success of much larger places, including Taiwan and Australia, in pursuing the same strategy. It also ignores the two enormous stimulus packages the state received from the federal government to support the economy through a prolonged downturn. Whether you compare the state as a whole to Kauaʻi (population 70,000) or to Australia (population 25 million), you reach the same conclusion: An island that controls its border, enforces a quarantine, and demonstrates competent public health resources can eradicate—not just "live with"—a deadly respiratory virus.

While it's tempting to judge the Honolulu establishment for these decisions, a harsh verdict would not be entirely fair. Much was done by both city and state that made a positive difference in the outcome. The early shutdown order by Caldwell in March, as well as the fourteen-day quarantine initiated by Ige, were critical moments. Delay by even another week or two would likely have led to hundreds, if not thousands, of additional deaths. Their action in advance of that crisis stands out in contrast to their counterparts on the Mainland. Not only that, but the government maintained these intrusive interventions for months. If someone had told me in early March 2020 that Hawaiʻi would soon turn off tourism, voluntarily, and keep it turned off until October, I would have thought that was an impossibility. But that's what the state did, and its eventual reopening, though imperfect and controversial, nonetheless included protections that were more rigorous than other states.

Caldwell and Kim also stood up public health infrastructure, going well beyond the usual role of mayors in Hawaiʻi, to fill gaps in the state response. These efforts were in their nature imperfect bandages, but by addressing deficiencies in the state response, they improved the safety of their counties.

There was opposition to all of this. Elements within the Oʻahu business community insisted on—some even sued for—the right to do business in ways that would have made the epidemic more deadly. Money was constantly pitted against lives, and as on the Mainland, a large and vocal minority preferred money. Physicians and public health officials had to resist these arguments and hold politicians accountable for the human outcome. And during the time when the threat was greatest, the politicians listened.

Each task the state undertook to reduce the severity of the epidemic, from imposing the quarantine on transpacific travelers to improving the scale of its contact tracing, required overcoming the voices that said such decisions were impractical or impossible. And yet the state did them, saving the lives of thousands of its residents. This indicates that fatalism was a self-fulfilling prophecy, and that the failures Hawaiʻi tolerated in the epidemic were cruelties it imposed on itself.

The state needs an honest conversation about the underlying causes of its shortcomings during the COVID-19 pandemic. In the absence of that reckoning, there's no guarantee that elected officials will be more adept at disease control next time than they were this time. They could easily be worse. Had Honolulu fared as poorly as Los Angeles, the city would have experienced over two thousand deaths, rather than three hundred fifty. If the state doesn't deal honestly with its dependence on tourism, and make adjustments to build its resiliency in the face of external shocks, then it's unlikely to improve its performance during future crises. Even between crises, the drawbacks of this dependence should be evident. It warps conversations about other priorities, such as preserving the environment for future generations, and it downgrades the relative importance of values like public education. The necessity of getting the tourism engine back online, even when it meant importing variant strains of virus, did not shine a flattering light on the state's leadership.

Given the economic benefits of tourism, and in particular the jobs it provides, no one should want that industry to fail. But debating tourism only as an economic discussion misses the point. The need to maintain a large visitor industry has consequences for the state's health. There's no guarantee that the next pandemic will be as benign as COVID-19. The world is entering a period of history in which it confronts not just unprecedented environmental degradation, but also a scientific age in which the ability to manipulate and engineer viruses exists in thousands of labs in dozens of countries. The next pandemic could be ten times as deadly as COVID-19, or ten times as contagious. It may well be a man-made pandemic. In such a scenario, Hawai'i will need to shut down its border, and possibly keep it shut down, while feeding and housing its residents. No one should assume that Hawai'i will be able to keep the tourism industry open at all during the next pandemic. Any economic discussion that doesn't account for this possibility is one that neglects the state's existential risks.

In every story there comes a time when the present must yield to the future. It's my hope that a descendant, an intellectual heir or a literal one, will find in this work encouragement to solve problems not yet imagined. Hawai'i is a small place, but its location and its people endow it with many natural advantages. In fighting the pandemic, the guardians of these islands cut with the grain of their geography and history. May it always be so for those who love Hawai'i best. ☙

AFTERWORD

September 2021

At a hospital in a rural area of Hawai'i, the staff thought they'd escaped the worst of the pandemic. The majority of patients, nurses, and doctors were vaccinated, and healthcare had mostly returned to normal. It was a half day for me, and I planned to see a few patients for minor ailments like wound infections and urinary tract infections. But that was the day the new SARS-CoV-2 variant arrived, and the small hospital transformed into a front line of the pandemic's most harrowing battle.

I sat and closed my eyes, trying to wrap my head around it. The infection control team had designated a wing of the building a "red zone," and they housed the positive patients there. Staff sealed the red zone with a plastic barrier, its only entrance through an antechamber next to the parking lot. Adjacent to the red zone was the "yellow zone," where patients exposed to known infections lived separately. The "green zone"—for the uninfected and unexposed—continued to function uneasily, and anyone entering for patient care took a rapid test.

As I reviewed charts, a test returned positive in the yellow zone. Nurses wheeled the patient into the red zone, which grew in size. I saw the humans retreat down the hallway, as the virus claimed an additional twenty feet of real estate.

I couldn't suppress a grim smile. The new variant had powers of transmission that commanded my respect. I suited up in the antechamber and visited the sick patients. Almost all of them were in their first twenty-four to forty-eight hours of symptoms, caught quickly by the alert doctors who staffed the wards. This was a novel experience. Typically I saw people admitted a week or two into their disease course, by which time it was too late to offer an effective anti-viral treatment. But here was a ward full of patients early in their course, exhibiting the first symptoms of COVID. I exited the red zone, and then I got on the phone. A few calls later, a car rolled up the Big Island coastline, carrying a precious cargo. I had never used monoclonal antibodies, and I'd assumed I wouldn't need them. But now we asked for the whole supply from the pharmacy.

Over the next week we treated the entire red zone, and then the yellow zone. Not a single patient deteriorated, and most never required oxygen. The virus that had advanced so rapidly down the hallway melted away as quickly as it had come. The sense of siege lifted, and was replaced with the exhilaration of a job well done.

A few weeks later I visited a new creation, one born of this success. The monoclonal antibody clinic at Queen's North Hawai'i is a virus deactivation engine. It is housed in a plantation-style building that used to be a cardiology suite. This was a minor disappointment. After my encounter at the rural hospital, I indulged grandiose visions. I asked Queen's for a tent, in order to scale up the treatment. I imagined something posh and cinematic, like Alexander on the march. But the facilities crew decided a building would do better in the Kamuela weather, and its location separate from the main hospital proved another advantage.

The aesthetic is nondescript, with a parking lot entrance leading to a lobby, marked by a sign that reads "Antibody Infusion Clinic." Inside are three rooms, each repurposed with an exhaust fan to produce negative pressure. The clinic welcomes the most contagious patients, and its nurses can administer up to a dozen infusions per day. The medicine consists of two manufactured antibodies that target different parts of the SARS-CoV-2 spike protein. This double hit retains effectiveness against variants. If given early in the disease course to a high-risk patient it can knock the infection out, sparing the hospital an admission and sparing the patient's life.

We are using monoclonal antibody treatments not only in the clinic, but in our emergency rooms and nursing homes. We are even beginning to use them subcutaneously in people's homes. It's the first direct antiviral therapy I've accessed that works. But it needs to be given early. Many people still don't receive the treatment, and Queen's is working to expand infrastructure and make it more widely available. I'll take what help I can get. Pulled back into the pandemic, I'm eager to try anything that tilts the balance back in our favor.

The late wave, Hawai'i's biggest, drowned the state's optimism, coming after the vaccine rollout and the long-delayed reopening of society. The wave consists almost entirely of the delta variant. Twice as contagious as the original strain, and with a viral burden a thousand times higher, delta has spread around the world and become the dominant strain of SARS-CoV-2. We're now confronting an epidemic more contagious than smallpox, one that can race through non-immune populations and overwhelm hospitals even in places where 60 percent of the community is vaccinated. This has led to increased breakthrough infections in the vaccinated, which now account for up to 20 percent of total infections. Vaccinated people are still protected from hospitalization and death, but 10-15 percent of admissions are vaccine breakthrough cases, mostly amongst the immune suppressed and frail elderly.

How did we get here? Why are we forced back into the shadows after struggling so mightily to enter the light? This seems to me the most salient question.

Having struggled with my own disappointment, I can identify a few factors. One is the virus itself, which always had a say—perhaps the dominant one—in how the pandemic would progress. Given our inability to vaccinate the world in early 2021, the virus had ample time to evolve. The delta variant, which came from India, evolved in the context of uncontrolled spread through a population of over a billion people. Its transmission became so efficient that it behaves almost like a new disease.

But that doesn't tell the full story, and it doesn't explain why Hawai'i in particular now struggles under a greater disease burden than at any time during the pandemic. For those answers we need to look in the mirror. When the vaccine program began, there was great optimism and a natural desire to return to normal. The City and County of Honolulu jettisoned its tier system, so painstakingly arrived at. The other counties largely followed. The state never developed rapid antigen testing at scale, though more forward thinking countries like Germany have made excellent use of them, and in Hawai'i they would be particularly helpful for securing travel and schools. Border control became even more lax, with vaccination accepted as a substitute for testing. Kaua'i ended its mandatory fourteen-day entry quarantine, and the Big Island abandoned post-arrival testing. A massive increase in travel, coupled with inadequate testing and no restrictions on gatherings, created fertile ground for the new variant.

All of this shows a lack of wisdom. It shows how lazy political habits lead reliably to a bad outcome. And that draws me toward the final observation, which is that hundreds of thousands of adults in Hawai'i, and tens of millions in America, rejected vaccination, which was the single best tool for ending the pandemic.

The stalled vaccination program is the saddest example yet of the country's appetite for conspiracy leading to the needless deaths of thousands of people. For most who refused the vaccine, it was fear fed by confusion. For some it was part of an ideology of loathing directed at academia, corporations, or the government. And for many it was also an expression of group identity. Whatever the gateway, once you enter the anti-vax space, you encounter a house of mirrors, with misinformation that's perfectly tailored to your tastes. This isn't hippies on the corner ranting about mercury. The current state of anti-vax propaganda is polished and professional. People with seemingly sterling credentials make dramatic claims in well-produced videos. Non-falsifiable arguments—presented as reasonable concerns—are published in fake journals, with fake references. In a few hours, a worried mother can be reduced to a confused muddle, while being made to feel like she's uncovering profound and forbidden truths. And this is how, without meaning to, America embarked on the largest science experiment in the history of the world. Half the population received the vaccine. The other half randomized itself to the Middle Ages.

It's an unnecessary experiment, because we had three good clinical trials, which enrolled tens of thousands of people, and told us that the vaccines were safe and effective. We then had a number of confirmatory studies in the months following the deployment of the vaccines around the world. These data were mostly retrospective, but they benefited from their heterogeneity, and gave confidence that the result was reproduceable in a variety of different settings. The second round of data was as "real world" as science gets: healthcare systems in California and Texas, public health data from places like the United Kingdom and Israel. And for those with a more visual bent, the shape of the epidemic curve played out right in front of our eyes, every day, with deaths falling in each country that rolled out an mRNA or Adenovirus vaccine program.

But we are running the experiment anyway, with the dogged fanaticism of people who won't concede a point. And the results show a bloodbath among the unvaccinated, who now account for almost all COVID deaths. For those who are unvaccinated, 2020 lives on indefinitely, but with an even nastier virus. For the rest of us, it's like watching a horror show, as neighbors caught gazing at their online reflections fall ill and fill up the hospitals. In fact, if this was a real experiment, we would stop it for being unethical.

The hospital during the delta wave is a surreal experience. The unvaccinated patients who fill half the beds hold their religious totems, ingest their silver or zinc, and quote me their gurus. Ignorance now compromises the medical care of the entire town. It's like rounding in the fourteenth century.

I have negative feelings about this. When the virus first arrived in Hawaiʻi, I took my turn on the wards, and I've taken it since. I'm proud of that. But now we've entered the "optional phase" of the pandemic, as a friend so nicely put it. I'm not proud of that. I'm disappointed, and I feel let down that part of the state watched doctors and nurses put ourselves at risk for a year, only to choose to rerun the whole awful spectacle.

At some point we'll pause this experiment. We'll stop these people from killing themselves, and we'll stop them from taking some of us with them. Protecting kids—many still too young to vaccinate—will be a major impetus. It's already beginning to happen, as the FDA moves toward full approval of the vaccines, and industries from healthcare to sports insist that their people are safe to be around. Mandates may be unpopular, but they're the right thing to do for any business that wants to stay in business. There's no freedom to spread disease, or to overwhelm hospitals with it, and there never has been.

At some point we'll decide enough is enough. But that will all take time, and before it's over we will have the images of yet another self-inflicted wound to remember this pandemic by. ☙

BACKSTORY

The Backstory contains my thoughts on the pandemic as they developed in real time. Many of these entries originally appeared as Facebook posts. They show my reactions to events covered in the book, but without the benefit of hindsight. I include them as a way to keep myself honest, and as an opportunity to revisit topics of interest in a level of detail that might distract from the chronological narrative of the book.

The reader may wonder what benefit I derived from initiating these conversations online. That's a fair question that I asked myself on a few occasions. Not every post led to productive interactions, but I was surprised by how quickly my Facebook page became a forum for civil conversation on the pandemic. Many colleagues in the medical, legal, education, and business professions took these posts in the right spirit, as an opportunity to dialogue and to improve our thinking on a subject.

The posts, as well as a few associated documents I produced with colleagues and include here, form a congruent narrative of the pandemic in Hawaiʻi, one that I hope enriches the reader's appreciation of what it's like to navigate uncertainty in a medical emergency.

FACEBOOK, FEBRUARY 29, 2020

Coronavirus: Is It Overhyped?

There seems to be a lot of confusion about this, so it's a topic worthy of a deeper look.

When confronted with a new problem, most people have a bias towards their initial reaction. We look for data points that confirm our view and reassure us that we are reading the situation correctly. We also tend to be biased towards the status quo.

What was my initial bias towards coronavirus? That it was being overhyped. In infectious diseases the discovery of new infections is increasingly common, both because our population has grown and become more global, and because we have increasingly powerful tools to detect and describe new pathogens.

That means it's hard for me to get too excited by a new bug. When Ebola re-emerged a few years ago I was interested but honestly didn't spend too much time on it. I had actual patients with other infections to worry about, and I judged (correctly) that the risk to the United States was low. And those powerful new tools also reassured me. We had this novel coronavirus sequenced almost as soon as it was detected. Vaccine development is happening at a pace that was unimaginable when I was a child.

But as I paid more attention to the new virus, my hot take began to chill. I want to explain why, and what data points I am looking at. It's not going to be possible to get everyone to agree on what the actual threat level is. But the less confused we are about the parameters, the more useful the discourse.

The first thing that worried me was the data on transmission outside China. The situation in China is bad, but interpreting what's going on there is hard (at least for me) because of the chaotic nature of their situation. Case definitions have changed more than once. Resources in Wuhan were stretched to the breaking point. And the government has a media narrative (aka propaganda) that it is pushing.

So in order to un-confuse myself, I ignored the China data and began reading the part of the daily WHO report that deals with non-China infections. And if you read those reports, you see that even weeks ago there was community transmission occurring in neighboring countries. Not much. A few cases here and there in places like Singapore, Malaysia, and Japan. That trickle of cases was alarming, because it indicated that containment measures were not succeeding.

Next I defined for myself what would indicate a serious threat. The parameter I came up with was a logarithmic increase in non-China cases, particularly if that occurred over a relatively short time scale (i.e., a couple weeks, the expected latency period of the virus). When the Korean outbreak began in earnest in late February, and we started seeing additional clusters in Italy and Iran, that criterion was fulfilled.

That's when I stopped reassuring people. And that's when I found myself becoming frustrated by confused comparisons of the new virus with other infections, many of which (failing to account for the high rate of transmission) were intended to downplay its significance. I think the people speaking this way—some of them doctors—were well-intentioned. But I also think they weren't paying attention.

If you look at the measures being taken in countries heavily impacted by the new virus in order to control it, what you see is a level of disruption that few people alive are accustomed to. Prolonged closures of public spaces. Quarantines of entire towns. A massive decrease in air travel and public transit. What this amounts to is a major disruption in cultural and economic activity. And those measures seem to be slowing, but not stopping, spread of the virus.

It's not the apocalypse, but it's not normal life either.

So my level of worry is correspondingly high, and I think the data supports that.

Now that said, in order to keep myself honest, I should define once again what would change my mind. What needs to happen to convince me that this is being overhyped?

I can think of two big data points that are worth tracking. One is the fatality rate of the infection. If we find out that there's a massive number of barely symptomatic cases we are missing, and the true fatality rate is much lower than has been reported (i.e., 0.1 percent, as opposed to 2 percent) that would be reassuring. That would be mortality that's actually more on par with a flu season. A bad deal, but not as alarming as the current numbers suggest. (And I should point out that we don't yet have good data on mild or asymptomatic illness, so I expect some revision down in the fatality rate.) This scenario is possible, though a pandemic of a new virus with flu-like mortality would still be a big deal.

The other reassuring data point would be a decrease in transmission. Ebola was highly fatal, but I didn't worry much about it because the likelihood it would spread far without detection was low. If I see a similar pattern with coronavirus (i.e., containment is successful and the non-China cases begin to drop), that too will be soothing. But on this front the minimally symptomatic cases actually work against us (and may well be why containment has been failing).

Right now I am not seeing either of those data points shift dramatically, which is why I think the only responsible advice to give people is to prepare themselves for a significant disruption in ordinary life. A pandemic with a mortality of even 1 percent would be a very big deal. Which means that vacation you want to take is not as important as making sure you don't become a vector for someone's aging mother. Telehealth and tele-education should boom right now. Netflix should do a brisk business. And helping each other through an emergency is more important than pursuing our usual pleasures and ambitions.

FACEBOOK, MARCH 17, 2020

Coronavirus—What an Uncontrolled Outbreak Would Look Like

There's an argument circulating that because COVID disproportionately kills old people, we should focus our efforts on protecting the elderly and allow life to continue as normal for everyone else. One version of this was featured on Fox News and goes against the recommendations of Anthony Fauci, the leading infectious diseases expert at NIH, for aggressive social distancing. I'm also running into variations of this argument, e.g., lockdowns are totalitarian, they're unnecessary, etc. Here in Honolulu, many people are continuing to congregate in places like malls as if nothing is happening, and up until today we were still welcoming tourists.

It probably won't surprise anyone that I agree with Fauci, not Fox News. But I think it's worth unpacking these arguments a bit, because the cost of shutting down our social and economic lives—even if it's just for a month or two—is obviously big. This is painful, and we need to be real about that. Why can't we just cordon off the nursing homes and allow this virus to make its run?

Here are some numbers to consider from Honolulu, where I live. If you live elsewhere you can check the census website and run your own version of this equation, and feel free to substitute in more or less optimistic numbers. If there are epidemiologists reading this, I'm open to any comments you have. Keep in mind I'm a clinical ID doctor, and I'm relying on other experts for many of my assumptions here.

Honolulu County Population—980,000
Population over 65—17.7%
Population under 18—27.5%

We're younger in Honolulu than I thought! We'll leave kids out of this for now. And we'll adopt the approach of allowing transmission amongst middle-aged adults. We'll assume we are completely protecting those old people. That leaves us with 537,040 people in the middle-aged range who we are going to allow to be fully exposed to this virus, because no one wants to be broke.

Now let's assume Marc Lipsitch, the Harvard epidemiologist, is correct, and 20–70 percent of the population will become infected if transmission follows an uninterrupted pattern. We're not social distancing in order to keep the economy humming, so we could be on the high end of that estimate. But to give this argument it's best chance, I'll use the 20 percent number. That's 107,408 middle-aged people who become infected.

Next let's make some estimates about case fatality. Numbers here are all over the place. The Koreans are doing the best, and also have a young population. Their fatality rate as per the WHO is 0.9 percent. Most other countries are much higher. But let's assume we do better than the Koreans. We successfully cordon off all of those old people (not possible, but we do it). We will assume a rosy mortality rate of 0.5 percent in this scenario. Where does that leave us?

It leaves us with 537 dead people between the age of eighteen and sixty-five. These are people in the prime of their lives, many of whom are parents, and who fill critical roles in our community.

To put that number in perspective, Queen's Hospital (the biggest in our county) has approximately five hundred beds. That's the entire hospital. ICU beds are a tenth of the total. Each of those 537 people will require an ICU bed and—based on data from COVID in other places—will take between two to three weeks to die. We also have to consider the people who will require ICU beds and recover. That's likely to number in the thousands. Hospitalizations that use regular beds may well be in the tens of thousands.

Keep in mind this is an optimistic scenario, with low mortality assumptions, in which we assume we can completely protect the elderly and only have 20 percent of our middle-aged population infected despite partying on like it's 2019.

Now you can see why the virus has crushed cities, including places with modern healthcare systems. This is why every town where it takes a bite ends up completely shutting down, even if initially there is intense resistance to that idea.

When a hospital is overrun with contagious patients to the extent we are talking about above, it ceases to function as a normal hospital. It becomes a COVID hospital. The staff begin to fall ill as infection control becomes impossible, and patients with ordinary illnesses don't get treated.

This is how epidemics can become mass mortality events.

I share these thoughts because I want to throw some cold water on the notion that we can just cordon off the old people and expect a decent result. A high level of distancing will be required to slow the pace of the epidemic, if for no other reason than to ensure our hospitals remain safe. The trick will be to strike the right balance between epidemiology and economics. That's a real trade off, and it's not going to be easy. I hope the governor is surrounding himself with experts in both those fields to help him navigate the coming months.

I also hope we can change some of the basic assumptions I am making above by finding treatments that impact the course of the disease. Drugs that lower COVID severity could make a big impact. More rapid testing may allow us to remove contagious people from circulation without having to shut down everything. Heavy production of N95 masks and other protective gear will make the hospitals safer.

But so far we have done none of those things in the United States. We can't get people tested, we don't have enough masks for healthcare workers, and we're being rocked by supply shortages. In other words, we're functioning on the level of a developing country, and that's why Fauci is giving the advice he's giving.

FACEBOOK, MARCH 25, 2020

Coronavirus—What Winning Looks Like

The country, and much of the world, is shutting down public spaces in an attempt to limit the spread of the virus. But this strategy has obvious costs. Those costs are going to mount with time. "Shut it down" is a defensive strategy. It's the equivalent of covering our heads during a barrage of punches. In the long run, if it's the best we can do, it will be a loser's strategy. So let's talk about what winning against a pandemic looks like.

I'm going to make a couple assumptions that I hope we agree on before outlining what I would like to see happen. It's important that we use the same ground rules, so that we can argue cogently about specifics.

First, I'm going to assume that prolonged, large-scale unemployment is unbearable. At a certain point we need to let people out, because if we don't, we're looking at a Great Depression–scale economic crisis. Even if prolonged unemployment is the right move epidemiologically, it will lose support politically. So that means "shut it down" has to be temporary, or at least intermittent.

Second, I'm going to assume that we all want the hospitals to work when our family members need them. I'm not talking about ideology here. I don't care if we choose a private or public model for solving a given aspect of this crisis. (I'm actually irritated by point scoring on this topic, as the failures in both our public and private systems should be clear to anyone who is being honest.) Let's put the politics of healthcare aside. I'm just stating that we need the system to work. The hospitals can't become movie sets from zombie films. They have to provide effective care, and they have to be safe to visit. And that means we have to avoid having them overrun by ill and contagious patients.

Those two requirements are currently at odds with each other, and that's the essence of our problem. Even worse, there's no quick escape from the tension. The best way out of this trap is a vaccine, but that's a year away. We have to survive during that time, and we have to get the upper hand on this epidemic before the vaccine arrives.

In order to accomplish that, we need a strategy for rapidly identifying who is sick and who is not. We need to see the virus in order to counter it. And this brings me to an approach that some bright epidemiologists have been pushing for months, which is to dramatically expand testing capacity. Currently in the United States, testing is for sick people who meet certain criteria. The criteria change almost daily and by location. That's because of severe resource limitations. Testing is also for celebrities and politicians, who don't yet seem aware of the stigma that will be attached to their line jumping in an emergency.

But the most alert scientists want us to change our entire relationship to testing. First a little historical overview. PCR-based lab tests emerged as a research tool decades ago. Around the time of the swine flu pandemic in 2009, they became common in hospitals, replacing the traditional influenza tests. In the past five years or so, "multiplex" PCR tests that look for dozens of bacteria or viruses with a single swab have become available. At my hospital we now routinely use multiplex tests to find the cause of respiratory infections, meningitis, and diarrhea. But the tests come attached to a steep bill, which in turn has led to concerns about over-testing. They have remained the province of internists and other doctors caring for seriously ill people.

That's the model we need to break. In the new model, a PCR test is for anyone who thinks they need a test. In the new model, the doctor is not a gatekeeper. The doctor is not even involved until there's a result to review. And that's because the reason to test isn't about an individual patient visit. Rather it's about infection control on a population scale. We need to know who is infected so we can get them out of circulation. Telling everyone with a sniffle to stay home will fail, especially as the economy erodes. And people who go out into public spaces need the confidence that those spaces are safe.

Trevor Bedford, a virologist at Fred Hutchinson, has outlined this strategy in some detail. It involves a massive surge in testing capacity. He calls it "the Apollo program of our time." But it's more than just increased testing. It is testing married to informatics. In this model a person has their test, and within a few hours they can access their result on a website or a phone app. The software provides them with useful information on what to do next, including instructions on how to self-isolate. It coordinates any e-prescriptions needed. It arranges a telehealth meeting with their doctor. It even assists them in contact tracing and notification if they are COVID positive. The traditional system of manual testing and follow-up with the Department of Health becomes largely automated, and that human time is reserved for people who don't have access to computers or who require special attention.

A system based on a massive (and smart) expansion of testing allows us to open up society. Something like normal life can happen without an unexpected wave of illness striking.

This won't be perfect, but it doesn't need to be. If we look at countries like Korea that embraced this approach early, they're still having new cases every day. But because they have interrupted transmission of the virus, those cases are a small fraction of what's happening in Europe and the United States. It's also a lot cheaper than shutting down the entire economy. In Korea they have tested less than 1 percent of their population. To put that in context locally, in Hawaiʻi it would be about twelve thousand tests (the current number is around three thousand five hundred).

The United States in general is late, and in places like New York, transmission is so widespread that testing now will have limited impact. But it will still be necessary when we emerge from "shut it down" and begin to open our public spaces. And cost should be no issue. The advantage of ramping up this technology is that the price per test will drop. Even if we had to test 5 percent of the population, and repeat that at regular intervals, we would be in a much better situation than we are now. To put it starkly, we can spend billions of dollars getting people access to good information, or trillions of dollars waiting to get punched.

There are other aspects to "winning" that are more intuitive. Healthcare workers need protective gear like N95 masks, and production of these should be ramped up logarithmically. Even if this happens, we are facing weeks of shortages, and we will have a number of dead doctors and nurses as a result. Anyone who is in the way of this effort for any reason should be discharged from their duties. The same goes for the effort to expand access to drugs and ventilators.

Even if we do everything correctly, we are looking at a prolonged period of social disruption. In computer models of the epidemic, ongoing social distancing is required to prevent large eruptions of cases. Until we have a vaccine, or become immune through a mass mortality event, we will continue to see periodic closings of our public spaces. Norms around social interaction may undergo long-term changes.

For me this feels like the end of an era. When I did antibiotic stewardship at Queen's, we had to deal with price gouging and periodic shortages of drugs. One odd feature of our global supply chains is that rather than making everything cheaper, as intended, they would often allow for petty monopolies and overcharging. The system was obviously broken but seemingly unfixable. What the pandemic is now showing us, as hospitals are overwhelmed and nurses are inadequately protected, is that this approach wasn't just a failure economically. It was a failure morally. The people who right that injustice, and restore our sovereignty over our health, will become leaders in this country.

FACEBOOK, APRIL 4, 2020

Coronavirus—I Am Dating Several Models

Just how screwed are we, precisely? That's an important question, and a lot of bright people are trying to answer it. It's no surprise to me that it was a model produced by Imperial College in London that finally cut through the fog of denial enveloping our politicians. That model predicted 2.5 million deaths in the United States if normal activities continued. But another model released by IHME shortly afterwards predicted eighty-five thousand deaths. The people working on that model were no less talented. How can there be a thirty-fold difference in mortality projections? And can we trust any model if the range between them is so enormous?

I ran my own model a week back, and it was enlightening. I used some software available through the University of Pennsylvania. It allows you to plug in local demographics and make assumptions about how the virus will behave. As I've discussed previously, there's huge debate over exactly how deadly the virus is and how much transmission is mild or asymptomatic. We also know that viral transmission depends on human behavior, and this variable fluctuates with time. This is a virus that loves spring break and packed Vegas casinos, but not lonely walks in the woods. All of these factors go into the models, which explains the huge spread of projections.

The key factor, in my view, is viral transmission. In the models you can assume a virus that's twice as deadly, and you'll get twice as many deaths. That's a linear relationship. But if you make the virus twice as transmissible, that has an exponential impact on your body count. That's because the virus is expanding through time. Under normal circumstances, cases double every three to four days. Anything we do to increase transmission is magnified through the population by shortening that doubling time. This is how you get a steep epidemic curve that overwhelms the healthcare system and creates a mass mortality event.

The differences between the models, then, boil down mostly to different assumptions about transmission. The bleak Imperial College forecast assumed we do nothing to stop transmission (they also included more optimistic projections based on different measures to reduce transmission). The IHME report assumed intense measures to reduce virus transmission. So the models aren't as much at odds as they seem. You plug in different assumptions, and the math of exponential growth is relentless.

In the end, it doesn't matter which model is right, because a model is only helpful if it tells us what to do. Which lever do we need to pull? We have no control over how nasty the virus is, though we will expend a lot of energy trying to pin that down. We do have control over transmission. That's good news, as it's the most important factor. So what the models have taught me is that we need to focus like a laser beam on viral transmission. That's the lever that—if pulled in a timely and effective way—will save millions of lives.

We're already impacting transmission through the intense social distancing that's now in place across much of the world. But a study of the places that have handled coronavirus well shows us that there are other ways to reduce transmission. Early and widespread testing reduces transmission. It's unbelievable to me that as recently as a week or two ago, people in the United States were still arguing that it's OK not to test people. That argument is over, and the body count settled it. Of course it's not the testing alone that makes the difference. It's testing merged with useful information to patients about self-isolation. It's contact tracing that identifies everyone associated with a positive test, and leads them to get tested. It's the establishment of effective quarantine than ensures mildly ill people don't infect their family members. Even universal masking is a strategy that's not intended to protect individuals, but rather to interrupt transmission.

Transmission is the enemy. Countries that understand that have adopted strategies to interrupt it. And this shows up clearly in their epidemic curves and in the number of people who die.

CIVIL BEAT, APRIL 7, 2020

Hawai'i's Hotels Can Help Lead The Fight Against This Pandemic

by David Derauf and Jonathan Dworkin

Hawai'i's tourism industry has the unique, time-sensitive opportunity to help the state contain the spread of COVID-19.

Hawai'i is at a disadvantage in resources compared to many places, but we do have a superabundance of unused hotel rooms at present. These are sunk costs for the hotels, but they are worth gold to doctors and epidemiologists.

There are two ways in which the state can mobilize these rooms—and the staff that service them—to help control the epidemic locally.

First, we know from the experience of other countries that doctors, nurses, and EMS technicians are infected at a high rate. That leads to secondary spread among their families at home. Getting frontline healthcare workers out of their houses is an urgent priority to knock down the epidemic.

Recent news that hotels are being made available for frontline workers (Hotels for Heroes) is a great start! Each island, as well as remote communities like Hāna, should designate at least one such hotel where physicians, nurses, and first responders can reside while doing frontline medical work with coronavirus patients.

Second, we should establish an "attentive care hotel" for asymptomatic and mildly ill patients.

Hawai'i leads the nation in multigenerational housing, and we are already seeing patients who acquired the virus at home.

National and international guidelines stress the need to isolate in a private bedroom and bathroom. For many families in Hawai'i that is not possible.

When patients are newly diagnosed, health officials should trace their contacts, and critically, evaluate their home situation. Those who wish to stay home while ill should do so.

But people who have legitimate reasons to worry they will infect a family member should be offered a room. With their own place to sleep and shower, the risk of secondary transmission in our community will drop.

The objection to attentive care hotel is that it would cause stigma for the hotel industry, but the opposite is true. The industry will suffer a far greater stigma if it doesn't help people while rooms sit empty and Hawai'i residents infect each other in overcrowded housing.

We know how to clean rooms where patients have stayed, and the virus does not survive long in the environment. A hotel that serves this function would require professional cleaning after a patient returns home, but it could return to normal business within days of the epidemic ending. FEMA funding can be made available to assist the quarantine effort, reimburse the hotel, and pay workers.

In previous times of crisis, Hawai'i's hotels participated in the common effort.

During World War II, the Royal Hawaiian was used by American troops. Even President Roosevelt famously stayed in Waikīkī during meetings with his Pacific commanders in July 1944. During the current epidemic, New York and San Francisco have mobilized their hotels to serve as quarantine facilities.

There's sound precedent—in history and in the present—for turning a tourist post into a command post and mobilizing the service industry to serve a higher cause.

In every model of this epidemic, the critical element that determines how many people die is the transmissibility of the virus. Anything we can do as a community to reduce transmission will have an outsized impact on lives saved. Failing to act early will bring us a higher body count.

We also know the American approach on transmission has failed so far. The CDC's centralized testing for the virus was so delayed that the epidemic took root unseen.

We have been slow to implement aggressive contact tracing, adopt protective equipment like masks in public, and develop an effective system of quarantine. In contrast, countries in East Asia have implemented all these policies and are now fighting an epidemic that's an order of magnitude smaller than ours.

The good news is that it's not too late for Hawaiʻi to avoid the large epidemic plaguing the Mainland, and our tourism industry is uniquely situated to help in that effort. It can do that by joining the governor's pandemic response team and making hotels one of our most effective assets against the virus.

FACEBOOK, MAY 3, 2020

COVID-19 and Fatality Rates

One of the big questions that I identified when I first asserted that COVID-19 is a big deal, and not merely a media event, is the fatality rate of the infection. To keep myself honest I said that if it turns out that it's much lower than previously expected, that would force me to re-evaluate my view of the situation.

To some extent this is now a moot point. Any epidemic bad enough to nearly overwhelm the healthcare capacity of a city like New York (despite a full lockdown) is *bad*, regardless of the ultimate calculated fatality.

But the question of fatality has nagged us throughout, and it has repercussions for how we think about opening up. It turns out it's a lot harder to answer than I initially expected.

First a few observations on why it's hard to get at:

1) We undercount deaths. There's excess mortality that's noticeable in death statistics that has not been attributed to COVID. Some of this is

due to COVID directly (i.e., undiagnosed patients), and some of it may be the indirect result of the shutdown. Those deaths lead you in opposite directions in regards to policy, and getting at this problem is difficult.

2) We undercount cases. The testing problems are severe and well described. It's likely that we have undercounted true cases of disease by a factor of ten to twenty times or more.

3) Serology studies are a mess. This was supposed to be how we get reliable data on the total number of people infected. But many of the early studies suffer from methodological problems in their sampling, technical problems in the performance of the test kits, and political problems from the results being immediately weaponized to push one agenda or another. Two of those three problems are being solved.

4) There's age stratification. The fatality rate is orders of magnitude higher in the elderly than in the young. But it can be deadly and debilitating in middle-aged people as well, and we're only just beginning to understand some of the clinical features (e.g., blood clotting problems).

So how do we make sense of all of this? First, by looking at a number of serology studies, we can correct in the flaws of any one method. When we look at data from different towns in Europe and the United States, most studies are showing an infection fatality rate of 0.3–0.7 percent. On the extreme ends are Santa Clara (0.1–0.2 percent) and NYC (approximately 1 percent).

That sounds pretty good, at least superficially. The number typically associated with flu is 0.1%. So our pandemic is three to seven times worse than flu. Put that way, maybe not so good. Even worse, it turns out that flu number itself is a bit fishy. If you count deaths directly attributable to flu (as we're doing with COVID), it's a lot lower. So the apples to apples comparison between COVID and flu shows an epidemic eight to ten times worse, possibly more.

That's certainly what it feels like from the healthcare provider side of things. Having worked through ten flu seasons, I never saw influenza fill up two units of our hospital with desperately ill people. And in Hawai'i we got lucky! But this is just anecdote. What we see in practice may have explanations that we don't yet fully appreciate.

For now, my best guess is that we're dealing with something five to ten times more fatal than flu, and likely a lot more contagious. Because there's no innate immunity, it can race through our population and cause a lot more illnesses than a typical flu season. These effects combined explain what we're seeing.

But I intend to remain open-minded on these points. We don't understand basic features of this epidemic in detail yet and that's why scientific discussions need some room to breathe, separate from politics, and prior to informing policy.

FACEBOOK, MAY 10, 2020

Hawaiʻi and COVID-19—The Circus at State

I'm one of dozens of people who signed a letter recently delivered to Governor Ige suggesting that he put in place stronger public health safeguards prior to opening the state. Other people signing included physicians, public health experts, and economists. The letter was channeled to Ige through members of Hawaiʻi's business community, who are worried about a failed reopening.

There's a tendency—intentional, I believe—to portray these concerns as being "anti-opening." The implication is that eggheads like us are just fine with lockdowns, because we are oblivious to the negative impacts they have on people's lives.

This is especially irritating to me, because when we first locked down I had an ominous feeling and even called it a "loser's strategy." Looking around the world, there are a few countries that avoided full lockdowns by making smart use of public health infrastructure. Interestingly, some of the best examples are islands, like Hawaiʻi. These are the people I admire, and their example (not the chaotic lockdowns that happened on the Mainland) is what informed the letter.

The problem with opening up in a dumb way, though, ought to be apparent. In order for the economy to meaningfully recover, people have to feel safe to participate in economic activity. Most people don't, because it's actually not safe. The president may be fine with two thousand deaths a day (that's ten airplanes crashing daily, over and over again) in exchange for some theoretical benefit in economic growth. But most people are going to decline that opportunity. So if we want the economy to come back for real, some competence in containing the epidemic is a prerequisite.

The Hawaiʻi letter calls for improvements in testing, increased staff for contact tracing, a strategy for isolation and quarantine of infected/exposed people, and special attention to high-risk groups where an outbreak could occur suddenly. This is all in lockstep with recommendations of national experts.

But Hawai'i residents probably won't be surprised to know that despite over a month of endless meetings, Hawai'i still hasn't delivered the goods here.

I'll offer some specifics. In regard to testing, we know that asymptomatic spread is particularly common in high-risk (i.e., overcrowded) situations. That means an outbreak can occur, with detection delayed, and then spillover can happen in the surrounding community. We're particularly concerned about nursing homes, public housing, and homeless shelters. We want those people tested, we want the workers tested, and we want regular access to testing. Nursing homes are of special concern, because while cases may begin asymptomatic, the ultimate mortality is high. There are also staff who work in more than one facility.

In Singapore, they had excellent control of COVID until an outbreak occurred in crowded workers' dormitories that they had neglected. They then jumped to one thousand-plus cases per day and were forced to lock down. That's what we want to avoid. The way to avoid it is to drop the self-destructive parsimony over testing, and give people access to the resource.

In regard to contact tracing, the best data suggests that to interrupt transmission it needs to happen early (ideally within twenty-four hours of case detection), and it needs to be comprehensive. This requires an ability to staff up quickly. The current Hawai'i DOH capacity is well below successful efforts in other countries. They say they don't need more help. But we want the governor to insist they have that help and are accountable for doing the tracing quickly and at scale. The COVID response can't be about respecting political fiefdoms. It has to be about getting the capacity online.

Isolation (for infected people) and quarantine (for exposed people) is another area where we are accepting bland reassurances rather than insisting on a robust system. We have a city full of empty hotel rooms, and there's now a plan on paper to use some of them if isolation and quarantine are needed. But based on several conversations I've had with state officials, I can tell you there's little appetite to do this. Most sick people will remain at home, even if there's no good way for them to self-isolate.

Ultimately the biggest obstacle in Hawai'i is not our limited infrastructure. It's the government's mentality of excuse making. And that's where the governor comes in. It's his job to make sure the state response functions as it should. It's his office that can break down the petty territorial fights between departments. It's his duty to hold people accountable for producing concrete goods rather than PR.

We all understand that state bureaucracy can be clunky. Under normal circumstances, we put up with some dysfunction. But the purpose of the letter is to clarify that normal dysfunction isn't good enough now. We need a system that actually works.

The best way—the only way—to bring back economic life is to make it safer for people to go out and interact. We can't spin our way out of that. We don't want some blue-state version of the White House here. It actually has to be safe, and people have to feel that.

So our appeal to Ige is a simple one. Get these things done, so life on these islands can begin to come back with some confidence.

CIVIL BEAT, JUNE 11, 2020

Public letter signed by more than 400 people, many in the healthcare sector:

The "Second Letter" to the Governor
by Jonathan Dworkin, David Derauf, Tim Brown, Chad Meyer, and Sumner La Croix

I Maluhia Kākou—A Plan for Opening Hawai'i Safely

May 27, 2020
Honorable Governor David Ige
Governor of the State of Hawai'i
State Capitol, Fifth Floor Executive Chambers
Honolulu, HI 96813

Aloha e Governor Ige:

The way to restore Hawai'i's economy is to prevent reintroduction of the virus.

Hawai'i continues to fare well in the coronavirus pandemic. This is in large part because airplane and cruise ship travel has been decreased by the fourteen-day quarantine order, and because residents have adhered to a prolonged and unsustainable shutdown of social and economic activity. Now we must find a way towards an economic revival that supports the people and their health.

In the eighteenth and nineteenth centuries, visitors to Hawai'i introduced many waves of infection that had a devastating impact on the health of the people. With that history in mind, and with our improved understanding of the science of how infections spread, we have an obligation to ensure that uncontrolled infection never again harms the people of Hawai'i.

Our goal should be to eliminate COVID-19 transmission within the Islands, while also taking steps to revitalize the economy and community life. As Hawai'i's economy is largely dependent on tourism, we must develop a plan to prevent the arrival of infected individuals. If we excel at this task and keep our infection rate low, we will attract responsible visitors who wish to enjoy the benefit of travel in a beautiful and disease-free state. Such visitors will expect to encounter extra steps during their trip to ensure that Hawai'i remains safe.

Specific Actions Recommended:

1. The state should develop a test-based strategy for preventing importation of new cases of COVID-19 through airports. Work on this should begin immediately, as visitor numbers at present are small, and it will take weeks to stand up a system that can function at scale.

2. The visitor strategy should include pretravel, test-based screening for air travelers to reduce the risk that they are infected with COVID-19 before interacting with the local population. Many patients are infectious before symptoms develop, and numerous studies have shown that temperature checks are ineffective as a primary means of screening. **Temperature checks and symptom screening are not sufficient to protect the people of Hawai'i** and will miss many infected patients. Quarantine policies should be maintained and enforced for travelers from endemic areas who don't wish to be tested.

3. Hospitality industry workers should be protected by this system, including regular access to testing and other healthcare services, as well as modified service protocols to protect them from travelers who test positive or refuse testing.

4. A more robust system of testing, contact tracing, isolation/quarantine, and surveillance must be grown. Expanded training of contact tracing personnel should be prioritized now, in anticipation of a summer surge in cases as tourism returns. Free, credited training programs such as the Johns Hopkins/Bloomberg program are available and can supplement state efforts. Work can also be done at the county level by having the Department of Health authorize experienced individuals to oversee program development and expansion. This rapid growth may require assistance from outside the Department of Health. The governor should expect cooperation from the different involved elements and accountability for meeting specific metrics. This should include timely (within twenty-four hours) and comprehensive contact tracing of all cases. Metrics of success should be monitored and publicly available to assess the efforts and to reassure the public that the system is functional.

5. Given the low number of cases currently circulating amongst the local population, the state should lift stay-at-home orders and allow for increased ease of travel between islands. High standards of respiratory hygiene should be maintained, including wearing masks in crowded areas and maintaining spacing. Sick people should not be allowed to board airplanes.

6. The state should continue to coordinate with county mayors who are initiating a phased reopening of businesses, with lower-risk businesses reopening first. The effort should be paired with disease surveillance, so that people have confidence that the reopening is occurring in a way that's safe and sustainable. Higher-risk businesses that require significant modifications to reopen should receive financial support for renovations from the county and state disaster relief funding.

7. One of the greatest risks as we open up is "superspreaders," large transmission events linked to infected individuals and facilitated by crowded gatherings that do not follow physical distancing. Gatherings of more than ten people should continue to be restricted to limit the size of any outbreaks. Gathering size limitations should be revisited every two weeks if case counts remain low and the state builds an effective system to prevent importation of new cases.

8. Medical practices and hospitals in Hawai'i should resume routine patient care, but with elevated precautions in place to separate potential COVID-19 patients from other patients. In particular, primary care and outpatient offices should continue to make use of symptoms-based screening prior to visits and enhanced use of telehealth.

9. Effective messaging to medical professionals and to the public at large should be a priority. In order to build trust, limitations in the state response so far should be acknowledged, with a plan outlined to improve performance and integration of the various state agencies. Culturally appropriate messaging should be used to reinforce concepts like crowd avoidance and respiratory hygiene with the public.

10. Mask wearing in crowded public spaces and in public transportation should be required in order to increase adherence. Hand hygiene should be readily available in all public places. Messaging around mask wearing should focus on it as a social responsibility and way of showing respect for others.

Without delay, state leadership should:

1. Commit itself to a policy of eliminating transmission of COVID-19 in these islands.
2. Create a workable plan to verify testing of airplane passengers for COVID-19 prior to travel, with appropriate quarantine provisions for those who don't test or have evidence of illness.
3. Mandate the growth of testing, timely contact tracing, and quarantine services by the Department of Health and affiliated organizations that will work with them.
4. Establish clear protocols for voluntary placement of COVID-19 patients who cannot self-isolate at home into a quarantine facility. This includes use of specific hotels, safe cleaning criteria for those hotels to protect workers, eligibility criteria for admission, and wraparound services (e.g., medical check-ins, food delivery) for patients.
5. Increase test-based surveillance of high-risk populations and living situations. This includes healthcare workers, hospitality industry workers, shelters, prisons, nursing homes, and public housing.

FACEBOOK, AUGUST 14, 2020; *STAR-ADVERTISER*, AUGUST 23, 2020

Hawai'i's COVID-19 Response Is a Disgrace; Time for Accountability

Some frank talk between Hawai'i's doctors and its state government is long overdue. Back in February, when the epidemic first slipped beyond China, I did what a lot of other doctors did. I looked for guidance from our department of health. What I found, unfortunately, was a lot of BS about how "the risk is low," delivered in the sedating drawl of our official press conferences. Not convinced by this, I began to chart cases outside China. It became clear quickly that the risk was not, in fact, low. I did my best to warn people at the end of February that bad things were coming at us fast.

And so I lost faith in official pronouncements before a lot of my colleagues. But I didn't become angry until a patient—a person who worked in tourism—began coughing. I was refused a COVID test by the DOH. Why? Because the patient hadn't traveled to a "high-risk" area. I pointed out that this was ridiculous, as there were already large epidemics happening in Korea, Iran, and Italy, with cases documented in numerous other countries. But our state officials stuck to their outdated policy, and I never did find out if that patient was infected. We now know that cases were circulating in the United States as early as January, and that testing restrictions allowed hundreds of people to become infected in secret. But what made me really mad was the thought of thousands of doctors and nurses exposing themselves every day to potentially infected people, and that our health department, rather than sticking up for us, was repeating a bunch of talking points. I try to be generous towards my colleagues, because I'm far from perfect in my own life. But I'm not a tool, and I still haven't forgotten this treatment.

When we were hit by the first wave a few weeks later, it became apparent that the DOH had no intention of ramping up its testing to anything close to a sufficient level, and their testing criteria remained inappropriately narrow. This wasn't a matter of being slow. It was a policy of minimizing risk and undercounting cases. The evidence is that for months now, even at times when capacity hasn't been a bottleneck, they have refused to test close contacts of infected patients.

What saved us in April was the effort of private labs, who ended up diagnosing the vast majority of infections in the Islands. And we were saved by drive-in testing, much of it organized by Scott Miscovich, whose blunt criticism of the state response made him a hated person in government circles. I have no doubt that without those private efforts, we would have been hearing "the risk is low" right until our ICUs filled up.

During the lockdown there was a lot of talk of successful reopening. But the problem was always the reliance of such an opening on our public health infrastructure. To have a successful reopening, you need to seek out the virus, trace contacts in a timely way, and establish effective isolation and quarantine. All of those are DOH functions, and the emergency response structure at HI-EMA should have helped them ramp up capacity. But none of this happened. This wasn't due to a lack of effort and communication. I have largely refrained from criticizing DOH and HI-EMA in public, as have most of my colleagues. This is because we were desperate (too desperate, I now realize) to understand them and work productively with them. We assumed, as decent humans do, that they must need help. But what we encountered was an impermeable wall of arrogance. No mistake admitted. No desire to be proactive. No transparency. No accountability. And the constant insistence that only they could provide core functions that they were, in fact, unwilling to provide.

We're now living with the consequences of that. It's become obvious in recent weeks that the contact tracing operation on Oʻahu isn't just inadequately staffed, it's qualitatively poor. There are marked delays in contacting people, and this was happening even before the surge in cases. People are infecting each other in crowded apartments while hotels sit empty. Close contacts are being refused testing by the officials responsible for testing them. And when the inevitable results of this callous system crashed down on a million residents of the Islands, what was the new talking point? That contact tracing isn't all that important after all. And that the people are to blame for not being attentive enough to state dictates.

Personal behavior does of course matter, and it hasn't all been good. But Hawaiʻi has done much better than the Mainland on this score. The vast majority of Hawaiʻi residents have supported every government effort to control transmission, including the ones that inflicted deep economic injury. This epidemic was zero to three cases per day in May, and that's because the people listened. A robust public health system would have eradicated COVID from these islands. A competent one would have at least allowed us to prevent it from doubling every eight to ten days. Instead we're looking at two hundred–plus cases per day, and that's with 90 percent of the tourism industry dead. The numbers here are staggering. There's no excuse for them. It's failure on an immense scale, and it can't be hidden or deflected.

But that doesn't mean we won't see an effort to confuse people. Even now, there's a veil of obfuscation. The latest ploy is to define down their responsibilities to the point where they become meaningless. "We don't test," is a recent refrain. Contact tracing also isn't their thing. And after six months, they haven't begun to mobilize hotel rooms to the point of being able to separate infected and uninfected people. What do you call a public health effort that doesn't test, doesn't contact trace, and doesn't quarantine? I can think of a few choice words, but none of them are polite.

The counties are now having to stand these services up in the face of an emergency, and they're right to do so. At least local government in Hawai'i—though imperfect—is trying to meet its responsibilities. But the state is another matter. In conversations I have had with state officials, I have been surprised—and I suspect the public would be, too—at how often it's just assumed that this virus will rip through the community. Losing isn't just acceptable to these people, it's a habit.

Many of us have asked pointedly and repeatedly to see basic metrics on the efficiency of DOH contact tracing. The former CDC director—whom they ought to respect if they don't respect ID doctors—has called for transparency from all state departments of health. But like students seeking to grade their own test, they want to define what is shared and what is kept secret. Even basic information on the location of cases remains obscure, crippling public awareness and the response of the counties, with patient privacy rolled out as the lame cover.

I don't know what else to do, other than to call it out. This is the opposite of science-based healthcare. Because science requires humility. It requires that you notice what works and what doesn't, and adjust your approach accordingly. It requires openness. It requires collegiality. It requires personal accountability. The state doesn't lack access to brains and talent. But our state bureaucracies worship control, and their administrators (I refuse to use the word "leaders") are critically short on these other qualities. What they're not short on is spin, excuses, and hostile redirection.

The governor, for his part, has been content to put up with this. He's aware of the shortcomings in the state response. I know that, because I've told him, as have numerous other doctors. But he's stood by his current team and allowed more talented individuals who work for the state to be ignored and silenced. The emergency structures he established have been crippled by many of the same personalities that made DOH ineffective. Ultimately it is the governor's job to break these impasses. The buck stops with him, and the full weight of this epidemic is now on his shoulders.

He may well be content to put up with it, or to shift around a few jobs while defending the broader failure. But I hope the people of Hawai'i—who are funding this wreckage that's now making them sick—stop putting up with it. We should all demand better. Because it's our goodwill, as well as our health, that the state has squandered.

FACEBOOK, NOVEMBER 29, 2020

Hawai'i Has a Safe Travels Program. So Is It Safe?

Since the pandemic began, no issue has been more contentious in Hawai'i than border control. And before I dive into the details of the state's Safe Travels program, I think it's worth noting that the arguments over tourism in many instances are not rational. There are times when these arguments seem to suck the oxygen out of the room. And yet what has actually killed us in terms of our virus response? Time and time again, it's the same activities. It's funeral and church services. It's gatherings at crowded housing units. It's lack of mask wearing and physical distancing between family, friends, and work colleagues.

I'm not saying border control isn't a worthy conversation. It's important and relevant. But to have an emotional argument about Waikīkī, while ignoring the repeated outbreaks related to our own activities, would be to miss the point. Let's not miss the point. Let's discuss tourism, but let's also keep it in perspective, and let's not let people off the hook in our local community who see spreading infection around as some kind of religious or economic right.

With that caveat in mind, it needs to be said that every island nation in the world that has done well during the pandemic has controlled its border. And unlike most other islands, we share a national boundary with the world's leading COVID idiots. Only in the United States has poor hygiene been made into a symbol of freedom. Only in the United

States do people routinely deny the basic facts of the situation, and express that denial as a kind of political grievance. So when we talk about tourism, we're talking about these people. We're talking about travel from a place with some of the highest COVID rates, and lowest adherence to public health recommendations, in the world.

In the local press right now there's a lot of argument about testing. But in my view, the original sin of Hawai'i's border control failure has nothing to do with testing. It has to do with quarantine. I remember some of the early conversations—back in March and April—about the establishment of the state's quarantine. And what became apparent at that time—and remains true now—is that the state had no interest in establishing a rigorous quarantine. The best way to see this is in reference to other countries. If you fly to Australia, you don't just fill out some papers in the airport and go wherever you want. Assuming your purpose for being there is deemed legitimate, you're assigned a hotel room. The government assumes responsibility for ensuring that no potentially infected person wanders around the community.

I emphasize this, because without an enforced quarantine, arguments about testing become abstractions. Whether it's no tests or ten, if people can show up and choose to "quarantine," and there's no attempt to ensure they actually do that, the whole system is predicated on a lie. The lack of enforced quarantine also makes it impossible to add layers of testing to the pretravel test, because visitors scatter in a hundred directions by the time you add the post-arrival layer. It becomes a logistical nightmare, rather than an added safeguard.

Quarantine, and the failure to enforce it, was the original error.

With that said, my colleague Darragh O'Carroll has written informatively about the advantages of two tests verses one. The basic point of a second test is to capture a second point in time. Two tests separated by five to seven days in time are a lot more likely to capture an infection, especially one in its early phases, than a single test. There have been arguments between bright people about how much more sensitive a second test is than a first. I'm going to leave that to the modelers, except to point out that we haven't studied this in humans in a prospective way, because that would require experimentally infecting humans. So much of the heat here comes from analyzing the effectiveness of various border control schemes, or reconstructing time-to-test positivity based on contact tracing of known cases.

This stuff is interesting, but what I find most compelling is our local data. And the data from Kaua'i tells us exactly how safe our travel program is. (See Figure 13.2, page 141.)

Tourism opened on October 15. Prior to tourism opening, Kaua'i had no endemic transmission. Now they have travel-related cases, and they are beginning to have community spread. It's not a large number of cases. But the difference between having COVID on your island, and not having it, is profound. In contrast, the other islands have seen increases in travel-related cases, but on islands like O 'ahu, where there is already endemic transmission, the travel introductions have been modest compared to the total, and overall numbers are stable.

What this tells me is that the Safe Travels program is providing some protection, but it's partial. The program benefits from the fact that most tourists don't interact intensively with locals, and that most locals wear masks. Presumably many of these travel introductions are dead ends. But on an island that had no endemic disease, you can see visually the burden that was added. And once a virus becomes endemic, your situation is fundamentally different. Normal activities, like school and local businesses, end up being impacted, and the disruption extends far beyond the tourism economy. You also begin to strain healthcare resources, and you begin to have deaths. As O 'ahu has shown, once the virus burrows in, it's very hard to get it out.

A major problem for the Safe Travels program has been the number of people who opt out of testing. Of the hundreds of thousands of recent travelers, about two-thirds received a pretravel test. Of the remaining third, a little more than half were deemed "exempt," and the rest chose to "quarantine." There are some additional details of interest. Of the travelers, almost a third were returning residents. And those returning residents were less likely to get a pretravel test. Less than half tested, and the rest were either exempt or opted to quarantine (presumably at local residences).

Putting this together, the problem is apparent. It's not just a matter of testing. It's that a sizable number of people are getting out of even one test, and a disproportionate number of them are locals who are far more likely to transmit virus to their families, friends, and co-workers.

So is the Safe Travels program safe? I'd say it's sorta safe. Maybe we should call it the "Hawai'i Sorta Safe Travels Program." We can serve free drinks on the flight, and everyone can reflect drunkenly on their mortality. The truth is that tourism is a bad business during a respiratory pandemic. No one at the state wants to hear that. But it's a point that's obvious to those of us who aren't up to our necks in local politics.

The good news is that we can make the program safer by insisting on a few modifications. The first would be to increase enforcement of the quarantine. That does double duty, because not only does it make it more likely people will test, but it gives you the capacity to add additional layers of protection later. For example, if you can enforce quarantine, you can shorten it by adding additional testing as needed. Another modification would be to eliminate the exemptions. The correct number of exemptions is zero. Doctors, nurses, security personnel, and other critical infrastructure workers should all be tested regularly in order to move freely. I also agree with adding a post-arrival test, and if resources are limited, I would prioritize returning residents and infrastructure workers, as these are the people most under-tested by our current system, and most likely to transmit infection.

Finally, we should allow counties like Kaua'i to adopt a more restrictive system if they deem it necessary. No island should be forced against the will of their mayor to accept endemic COVID-19 infection. That's an abuse of the relationship between the tourism industry and the people. And with a vaccine now on the horizon, those advocating that we need to accept casualties in exchange for economic activity have even less ground to stand on. Controlling the disease has always been the right approach. And no person on Kaua'i, or any other island, should die now in service of a misguided economic strategy.

FACEBOOK, DECEMBER 20, 2020

COVID mRNA Vaccines: Knowns, Unknowns, and Why I'll Get the Shot

The math of a pandemic is relentless. Given enough time, a large percentage of individuals will become infected, even with good adherence to public health practices. The whole point of listening to public health advice is to buy time. For what? For a better disease control strategy. That could be more rapid testing that allows us to stamp out transmission chains. It could be treatments that allow us to make the disease less dangerous. Or it could be a vaccine. For me, the vaccine always held the allure. You want to knock out a virus? You need a vaccine.

We now have multiple vaccines, but none are more intriguing than the first two going through the steps of FDA approval, issued by Pfizer and Moderna. They are similar, and I'd like to discuss them together. Both use a technology called messenger RNA. This didn't exist when I was in medical school, and I've had to familiarize myself with it the past year. The basic idea is to inject a molecule of messenger RNA into the muscle of a human. The mRNA does not integrate into human DNA. It is a temporary molecule, a genetic Post-it note, dwelling transiently in the cytoplasm of the cell. Its purpose is to tell the cell what protein to produce. Both vaccines use messenger RNA that encodes for the coronavirus spike protein. This in turn causes the muscle cells to produce the spike protein and trigger a protective immune response (both antibodies and T cells) against that virus surface protein.

It's a fairly simple idea, and the concept for this vaccine technology dates back decades. But it proved difficult to develop in practice because of problems stabilizing the messenger RNA long enough to do its job, as well as problems delivering it efficiently into the muscle cells. Early attempts used clumsy delivery vehicles and were chewed up so quickly by the immune system that they didn't stimulate a protective response. It's only in the past decade that the technology has become mature, and prior to 2020 there were no mRNA vaccines available in humans.

We now have two mRNA systems soon to be available to millions of people. How do we assess their safety and efficacy?

First, I think we need to acknowledge that because of the emergency we are living under, we were forced to compress the phase 2 and 3 trials into a shorter time period than is typical. I'd like to put this in context. When I attended the Infectious Diseases Society meeting in 2017, Anthony Fauci gave a speech on vaccine development. He pointed out that when SARS-CoV-1 was discovered in 2002, it took nineteen months to go from sequencing the virus to the first vaccine trial. By 2016, with Zika virus, sequence to first trial had been cut to three and a half months. This was stellar progress! But in 2020 we blew the previous records out of the water. We sequenced the virus in January, and by November we had completed not just initial but phase 3 trials.

That's an acceleration in vaccine development, but it's one that is consistent with the progress being made before the pandemic. I marvel at the achievement. But I'm not here to be a cheerleader. I want to know that the thing works, and I want to know that it will be safe when deployed to millions of people.

First there's efficacy. Both mRNA vaccines report high efficacy, 94 to 95 percent. That's much better than expected. If we experience that at scale, we can largely shut down the epidemic. But it's important to note that this efficacy was observed only over a couple months, and only looking at people with symptomatic infection. We don't yet know how long the protection lasts. We don't know if mutations in the virus spike protein will allow it to "escape" the vaccine, or how long that will take. We have little data about "severe" COVID, as there were only a few dozen patients in the trials who developed it. And we don't yet know much about viral shedding or transmission, though the Moderna study did suggest some benefit in reducing asymptomatic infection.

In other words, the efficacy data may translate perfectly to interruption of transmission. Or it may not. Until we know, we need to keep the masks on. Likewise we may get long-lasting immunity. Or we may not. We just don't know yet. We also don't know much about kids, pregnant women, or immune-suppressed patients.

None of that bothers me. Even if the mRNA vaccines contain some disappointments compared to their initial efficacy numbers, if they are anywhere close to 94 percent over a time course of a year, they will be by far our most useful tools to date. There are ongoing projects to clarify duration of immunity. Data on kids, pregnant women, and other select groups will be coming soon.

Now let's discuss safety. The most common effects are injection site pain, muscle aches, joint aches, headaches, fatigue, and fevers. These are "flu-like" symptoms. Coincidentally, this is what people experience when they complain that the flu shot "gives me the flu." They're not really side effects, because they're supposed to happen. The innate immune system is responding to the vaccine. This is a good thing. When this happens it's best not to take medicine like Tylenol unless you're miserable, as the immune response is exactly what you're going for. Better to watch some TV and spoil yourself with a bowl of soup.

But with the mRNA COVID vaccines, these innate immune responses are more intense than is typical. Some people are wiped out for a day or two. Many people have to take Tylenol to get comfortable. People should be warned they may feel lousy while their body mounts the immune response.

A larger issue than the innate immune response, however intense, is the potential for rare and more severe side effects. Because they have been studied in a few tens of thousands of people, we aren't yet aware of every potential adverse reaction. This is written clearly in the FDA documents. There's no attempt at subterfuge. But in the excitement over the vaccines, it's already being overlooked. I think it's a mistake to downplay this rhetorically. I won't be surprised if we find reactions that emerge only after we have vaccinated millions of people. These adverse reactions won't be very common (if they were, we would have seen them in the phase 3 data). But even a rare side effect, if unexpected and severe, will be a tragic occurrence. Doctors should speak plainly about it.

There's already some signal here. In the phase 3 data, allergic reactions were more common amongst vaccine recipients than placebo. Sure enough, there are case reports in the United Kingdom and the United States of nonfatal but serious allergic reactions in a few vaccine recipients. In the trials, seven patients experienced Bell's palsy, a paralysis of the facial nerve. That's fairly nasty, though often not permanent, and not considered life-threatening. Those seven patients were out of more than thirty thousand vaccinated. That's a low risk, but it appears higher than the baseline incidence of Bell's palsy. The numbers here are small enough that we can't be sure if it's a real association or just statistical noise. We will know more soon.

Some friends will argue that even by acknowledging uncertainty around the vaccine we are setting ourselves up for the inevitable cherry-picking and misinformation of the anti-vax movement. No doubt there will be individuals who will use uncertainty to stoke paranoia and service a political agenda. They will exaggerate any report of a rare adverse reaction, and downplay the risk of "natural" infection. Anything that goes wrong will be used in an attempt to pit us against one another. This is the lowest form of media. I have confidence in the people I regularly interact with to see through it, and counter it if necessary. Ultimately a process that speaks honestly about unknowns in science, and makes sure we address them, will be more trustworthy than one that fears propaganda spread by ignorant people.

I will take the vaccine as soon as it's available to me on the Big Island. And that's not a hard decision for me. In explanation, I should acknowledge my own biases. I examined the data for these new medicines in order to communicate honestly with patients and friends. But I also believe that the way to "win" in a pandemic is to crush transmission. And winning, not merely existing in a suspended society, is my goal.

Every time I enter a COVID room I think about my other patients. I think about my family. I don't want to get sick, but even more than that I don't want to be a vector and make other people sick. And I want us to emerge from this hellish year. We have sacrificed to control this disease, and now we have tools that may allow us to beat it. We can't simply avoid the virus indefinitely. Even on the islands that neighbor O'ahu, the virus will come. It's not reasonable to expect our mayors to permanently cut us off from the world, and they won't do it. The majority of us will either get a vaccine or get sick. And getting sick confers with it not just a risk of death, but the likelihood that we will transmit to others. Getting sick also involves far more problematic immune reactions than vaccination.

I was never a fan of "shut it down." In extremis, it was a means to this end. The end is the resumption of our lives, with the Islands protected. For that to happen, we don't have to suspend our skepticism. We should describe any warts in the data plainly. All that's needed for a healthy conversation is an acknowledgement of what's known and what isn't, alongside a reasonable weighing of risks and benefits. Reason hasn't been our strongpoint in 2020. But I'm hoping that this, too, changes with the new year. ☙

SOURCES

Introduction

O. A. Bushnell. *The Gifts of Civilization: Germs and Genocide in Hawai'i.* University of Hawai'i Press, 1993.

Robert Schmitt and Eleanor Nordyke. "Death in Hawai'i: The Epidemics of 1848–1849." Hawaiian Journal of History 35 (2001).

Sumner La Croix. *Hawai'i: Eight Hundred Years of Political and Economic Change.* University of Chicago Press, 2019.

Jen Krogstad. "Hawaii is home to the nation's largest share of multiracial Americans." Pew Research Center, Jun. 17, 2015.

Moises Velasquez-Manoff. "Want to Be Less Racist? Move to Hawaii." New York Times, Jun. 28, 2019.

Barack Obama. *Dreams from My Father: A Story of Race and Inheritance.* Times Books, 1995.

"Obama had multiethnic existence in Hawaii." NBC News, Feb. 6, 2007.

Catherine Rampell. "Discovered: The Happiest Man in America." *New York Times,* Mar. 5, 2011.

Hawai'i Visitor Statistics Released for 2019. Hawai'i Tourism Authority, Jan. 29, 2020.

"Monthly Visitor Statistics for 2019" page, Hawai'i Tourism Authority website.

Naome Akamine and Eugene Tian. *Hawaii's Working Population: An*

Analysis by Industry 2012–2016. Department of Business, Economic Development & Tourism Research and Economic Analysis Division.

George Szigeti. "Hawaii Tourism Set New Record Totals in 2017." The website of the Governor of the State of Hawai'i Governor David Y. Ige, Jan. 31, 2018.

Ku'uwehi Hiraishi. "It Takes Two: Faces of Hawai'i Workers With Multiple Jobs." Hawaii Public Radio, Sep. 3, 2018.

Stewart Yerton. "Has The Hawaii Tourism Industry Lost Its Clout?" Civil Beat, Dec. 2, 2020.

HTA Resident Sentiment Survey 2018 Highlights. Hawai'i Tourism Authority.

"ACT scores show most Hawaii students not 'college ready.'" Hawaii News Now, Aug. 24, 2016.

The Condition of College & Career Readiness 2018 Hawaii Key Findings. ACT Research, act.org.

Kathleen Gallagher. "UH resident tuition jumps 137% over past 10 years." Pacific Business News, Mar. 25, 2016.

Binsheng Li. *Hawaii Economic Structure Analysis Using the Industry Level Gross Domestic Product Data*. Department of Business, Economic Development and Tourism, July 2019.

Notes on interview with Sumner La Croix, Apr. 12, 2021.

University of Hawai'i Economic Research Organization (UHERO) Data Portal.

Ryan Finnerty. "Amid Calls For Diversification, A Look Back At Hawaii's History of Single-Industry Dominance." Hawaii Public Radio, Jun. 8, 2020.

James Mak and Justin Tyndall. "Aloha 'Oe: Population Migration Between Hawaii and the U.S. Mainland." UHERO, Aug. 6, 2020.

Natalie Schack. "A New Locally Owned Hotel Company." *Hawaii Business*. Mar. 11, 2019.

Ian Lind. "CMBS could pose risks for Hawai'i's hotels and retail properties." *iLind* (blog), May 6, 2020.

Private correspondence (e-mail) with Eric Gill, Local 5 union leader, Oct. 3, 2020.

Dan Frosch and Paul Overberg. "How a Train Through Paradise Turned Into a $9 Billion Debacle." *Wall Street Journal*, Mar. 22, 2019.

Courtney Cough et al. "Mass coral bleaching due to unprecedented marine heat wave in Papahānaumokuākea Marine National Monument (Northwestern Hawaiian Islands)." *PLOS ONE* 12, no. 9: (2017).

"Water Quality Data - Microbiology" page, Department of Health, Clean Water Branch website.

2018 State of Hawaii Water Quality Monitoring and Assessment Report. Department of Health, Clean Water Branch, Jul. 11, 2018.

Chapter One

Dennis Maki. "Emerging Infections." Chicago Board Review, Rush University, 2012.

Alexandra Levitt, Ali Khan, and James Hughes. "Emerging and re-emerging pathogens and diseases." *In Infectious Diseases*, edited by Jonathan Cohen, William G. Powderly, and Steven M. Opal, 58–59. Mosby: 2010.

"Nipah Virus - Transmission" page, Centers for Disease Control and Prevention website.

Elizabeth Thursby and Nathalie Juge. "Introduction to the human gut microbiota." *Biochemical Journal* 474 (2017): 1823–1836.

Miriam Barlow et al. "High Rate of Mobilization for blaCTX-Ms." Emerging Infectious Diseases 14, no. 3 (2008): 423–428.

Teresa Coque et al. "Dissemination of Clonally Related Escherichia coli Strains Expressing Extended Spectrum B-Lactamase CTX-M-15." *Emerging Infectious Diseases* 14, no. 2 (2008): 195–200.

C. R. Vitek and M. Wharton. "Diphtheria in the former Soviet Union: reemergence of a pandemic disease." *Emerging Infectious Diseases* 4, no. 4 (1998): 539–550.

Erica Hartmann et al. "Antimicrobial chemicals are associated with elevated antibiotic resistance genes in the indoor dust microbiome." *Environ Sci Technol* 50, no. 18 (2016): 9807–9815.

Richard Knox. "Origin of AIDS linked to colonial practices in Africa." National Public Radio, Jun. 4, 2006.

C. Heilmann et al. "Are coagulase-negative staphylococci virulent?" *Clinical Microbiology and Infection* 25, no. 9 (2019): 1071–1080.

Duane Gubler. "Dengue, Urbanization, and Globalization: The Unholy Trinity of the 21st Century." *Tropical Medicine and Health* 39 (2011): 3–11.

Jonathan Dworkin. "Emerging Infections: MERS and the New Normal." Queen's Medical Center Grand Rounds, July 2013.

Ming Wang et al. "SARS-CoV Infection in a Restaurant from Palm Civet." *Emerging Infectious Diseases* 11, no. 12 (2005): 1860–1865.

Obituary of Li Wenliang, *The Lancet*, February 18, 2020.

Nectar Gan, Caitlin Hu, and Ivan Watson. "Beijing tightens grip over coronavirus research, amid US-China row on virus origin." CNN, Apr. 16, 2020.

Edward C. Holmes (edward_holmes) on behalf of Yong-Zhen Zhang. "Novel 2019 coronavirus genome." Virological, Jan. 10, 2020.

Peng Zhou et al. "A pneumonia outbreak associated with a new coronavirus of probable bat origin." *Nature* 579 (2020): 270–273.

Jon Cohen. "Wuhan seafood market may not be source of novel virus spreading globally." Science, Jan. 26, 2020.

Rafi Letzter. "The coronavirus really didn't start at that Wuhan 'wet market.'" Live Science, May 28, 2020.

Personal correspondence with Dr. Alina Chan (Broad Institute), Oct. 16–17, 2020.

Jon Cohen. "Trump 'owes us an apology.' Chinese scientist at the center of COVID-19 origin theories speaks out." *Science*, Jul. 24, 2020.

Shi Zhengli. Reply to Science Magazine, *Science*, Jul. 2020.

Alina Chan (@Ayjchan). "Was RaTG13, the closest virus genome to SARS-CoV-2 (96.2% match), fabricated? …" Twitter, Sep. 18, 2020, 9:27 a.m.

Rowen Jacobsen. "Could COVID-19 Have Escaped from a Lab?" *Boston*, Sep. 9, 2020.

Nicholson Baker. "The Lab-Leak Hypothesis." *New York*, Jan. 4, 2021.

Giuseppina La Rosa et al. "SARS-CoV-2 has been circulating in northern Italy since December, 2019: Evidence from environmental monitoring." *Science of the Total Environment* 750 (2021).

Sridhar V. Basavaraju et al. "Serologic Testing of US Blood Donations to Identify Severe Acute Respiratory Syndrome Coronavirus 2 (SARS-CoV-2)–Reactive Antibodies: December 2019–January 2020." Clinical Infectious Diseases 72, no. 12 (2021).

Jonathan Pekar et al. "Timing the SARS-CoV-2 index case in Hubei province." *Science*, Mar. 18, 2021.

Josh Rogin. "In 2018, Diplomats Warned of Risky Coronavirus Experiments in a Wuhan Lab. No One Listened." *Politico*, Mar. 8, 2021.

Alina Chan (@Ayjchan). "I've been getting many questions about pre-Wuhan covid cases . . ." Twitter, Jan. 12, 2021, 5:16 p.m.

Matt Ridley and Alina Chan. "Did the COVID-19 Virus Really Escape From a Wuhan Lab?" The Rational Optimist, Feb. 7, 2021.

Alina Chan and Matt Ridley. "The World Needs a Real Investigation Into the Origins of Covid-19." *Wall Street Journal*, Jan. 15, 2021.

Bret Weinstein. "#65: Because Science (Bret Weinstein & Heather Heying DarkHorse Livestream)." ["Phylogenetic anomaly suggests lab origins," from 38-minute mark.] *DarkHorse Podcast*, Jan. 30, 2021.

Samantha Black. "How has SARS-CoV-2 evolved from bat coronavirus?" The Science Advisory Board, Jul. 9, 2020.

Bryan Johnson et al. "Loss of furin cleavage site attenuates SARS-CoV-2 pathogenesis." *Nature* 591 (2021): 293–299.

Maciej Boni et al. "Evolutionary origins of SARS-CoV-2 sarbecovirus lineage responsible for the COVID-19 pandemic." *Nature Microbiology* 5 (2020): 1408–1417.

"China delayed releasing coronavirus info, frustrating WHO." Associated Press, Jun. 2, 2020.

Jason Beaubien. "Why They're Called 'Wet Markets'—And What Health Risks They Might Pose." National Public Radio, Jan. 31, 2020.

China Opens First Bio Safety Level 4 Laboratory. State Department, Jan. 19, 2018.

Michelle Rozo and Gigi Kwik Gronvall. "The Reemergent 1977 H1N1 Strain and the Gain-of-Function Debate." *mBio* 6, no. 4 (2015).

"'Shabby' lab blamed for disease." BBC News, Mar. 11, 2008.

Alison Young. "Newly disclosed CDC biolab failures 'like a screenplay for a disaster movie.'" *USA Today*, Jun. 2, 2016.

Ian Sample. "Revealed: 100 safety breaches at UK labs handling potentially deadly pathogens." *The Guardian*, Dec. 4, 2014.

Simone McCarthy. "Coronavirus: WHO waits for China to approve pandemic origins investigators." *South China Morning Post*, Oct. 8, 2020.

Bill Birtles (@billbirtles). "Australian WHO #covid expert team member Dominic Dwyer . . ." Twitter, Feb. 10, 2021, 4:40 p.m.

Kai Kupferschmidt. "'Politics was always in the room.' WHO mission chief reflects on China trip seeking COVID-19's origin." *Science*, Feb. 14, 2021.

Emily Rauhala. "WHO Wuhan report leaves question of coronavirus origins unresolved." *Washington Post*, Mar. 29, 2021.

Amy Qin, Vivian Wang, and Danny Hakim. "How Steve Bannon and a Chinese Billionaire Created a Right-Wing Coronavirus Media Sensation." *New York Times*, Nov. 20, 2020.

Michael Gerson. "Opinion: The right is dwelling on slanderous myths about the origins of covid-19." *Washington Post*, May 24, 2021.

Glenn Kessler. "Fact-checking the Paul-Fauci flap over Wuhan lab funding." *Washington Post*, May 18, 2021.

Natasha Betrand et al. "New information on Wuhan researchers' illness furthers debate on pandemic origins." CNN, May 24, 2021.

Glenn Kessler. "Timeline: How the Wuhan lab-leak theory suddenly became credible." *Washington Post*, May 24, 2021.

Nicholas Wade. "The origin of COVID: Did people or nature open Pandora's box at Wuhan?" Bulletin of the Atomic Scientists, May 5, 2021.

Katherine Eban. "The Lab-Leak Theory: Inside the Fight to Uncover COVID-19's Origins." *Vanity Fair*, Jun. 3, 2021.

Alina Chan and Mark Lipsitch. "Why understanding the origin of COVID-19 is essential for policymakers: Discussing future regulations to prevent pandemics." Brookings video interview, 59:33, Jun. 7, 2021.

Chapter Two

"Coronavirus disease (COVID-10) Weekly Epidemiological Update and Weekly Operational Update" page, World Health Organization website.

Private correspondence (text and Facebook Messenger) with Masayuki Nogi, Feb. 16–25.

Paula Hancocks and Yoonjung Seo. "How novel coronavirus spread through the Shincheonji religious group in South Korea." CNN, Feb. 27, 2020.

Ahn Jun-yong. "Daegu in Lockdown as Coronavirus Infections Soar." *The Chosunilbo*, Feb 24, 2020.

Michele Senni. "COVID-19 experience in Bergamo, Italy." *European Heart Journal* 41, no. 19 (2020): 1783–1784.

Erin Cunningham and Dalton Bennett. "Coronavirus burial pits so vast they're visible from space." *Washington Post*, March 12, 2020.

Kristen Holmes, Nick Valencia, and Curt Devine. CDC woes bring Director Redfield's troubled past as an AIDS researcher to light." CNN, Jun. 5, 2020.

Rosalind Helderman. "After flight back to US, a growing number of Costa Luminosa cruise ship passengers have flu-like symptoms." Washington Post, Mar. 23, 2020.

Leah Moriart et al. "Public Health Responses to COVID-19 Outbreaks on Cruise Ships—Worldwide, February–March, 2020." *Morbidity and Mortality Weekly Report* 69, no. 12 (2020): 347–352.

Dan Diamond. "Federal turf wars over coronavirus rescues created 'health and safety issues,' watchdog concludes." *Washington Post*, Apr. 19, 2021.

HHS Should Clarify Agency Roles for Emergency Return of US Citizens During a Pandemic. Government Accountability Office, Apr. 2021.

Tamara Keith. "Timeline: What Trump Has Said And Done About Coronavirus." National Public Radio, Apr. 21, 2020.

Zubin Damania. Deadly Chinese Virus (Jan. 23, 2020), Coronavirus Update (Feb. 8, 2020), Coronavirus (with Peter Hotez, Mar. 1, 2020).

Trevor Bedford (@trvrb). "This is a thread about how to interpret the seemingly sudden appearance of #COVID19 across the much of the US . . ." Twitter, Mar. 13, 2020, 6:49 p.m.

Choi Jae-hee. "South Korea's best method of tracking COVID-19 spread: credit card transactions." *The Korea Herald*, Apr. 9, 2020.

June-Ho Kim et al. "Emerging COVID-19 success story: South Korea learned the lessons of MERS." Our World in Data, Mar. 5, 2021.

Kim Jaehan. "I got Coronavirus Test.. The result?" [Documentary of Korean quarantine system.] Facebook video, 6:57, Apr. 5, 2020, 6:21 a.m.

Private correspondence with David Derauf and Lin Xihong on South Korean COVID-19 measures, Mar. 28.

Anna Bonalume. "Devastated by coronavirus, did Bergamo's work ethic count against it?" *The Guardian*, Apr. 6, 2020.

Jason Horowitz. "The Lost Days That Made Bergamo a Coronavirus Tragedy." *New York Times*, Nov. 29, 2020.

Private correspondence with [retracted] on the recent scene from Qom Hospital, Mar. 3, 2020.

Muayad Merza et al. "COVID-19 outbreak in Iraqi Kurdistan: The first report characterizing epidemiological, clinical, laboratory, and radiographic findings of the disease." *Diabetes, Metabolic Syndrome and Obesity: Targets and Therapy* 14, no. 4 (2020): 547–554.

"Coronavirus Curfew Shuts Down Cities in Iraq's Kurdish Region." *Alsharq Al-Awsat*, Mar. 14, 2020.

Karwan Faidhi Dri. "Sulaimani 'will be another Italy' as COVID-19 resurges: governor." Rudaw, Jun. 6, 2020.

Idiris Okuduci et al. "Iraq's KRG eases coronavirus lockdown after two months." Anadolu Agency, May 12, 2020.

Zhelwan Wali. "Erbil eases some COVID-19 lockdown restrictions." Rudaw, Jul. 11, 2020.

Private correspondence with Hawar Mykhan, Feb. 11–12, 2021.

Jacinda Ardern. "Major steps taken to protect New Zealander's from COVID-19." The official website of the New Zealand Government, Mar. 14, 2020.

John Barry. *The Great Influenza*. Penguin Random House, 2004.

Nancy Tomes. "'Destroyer and Teacher': Managing the Masses During the 1918–1919 Influenza Pandemic." *Public Health Reports* 125 (2010): 48–62.

Chapter Three

Hawai'i Visitor Statistics Released for February 2020. Hawai'i Tourism Authority, Mar. 31, 2020.

"Monthly Visitor Statistics for 2020" page, Hawai'i Tourism Authority website.

Michelle Jorden et al. "Evidence for Limited Early Spread of COVID-19 Within the United States, January–February 2020." *Morbidity and Mortality Weekly Report* 69, no. 22 (2020): 680–684.

"Department of Health Steps up Testing for COVID-19: About 200 Tests to be Conducted Each Week." Department of Health, Mar. 10, 2020.

Personal correspondence (e-mail) to Erlaine Bello on COVID-19 preparedness and PUI definition, Feb. 25–26, 2020.

Personal correspondence (e-mail) with Erlaine Bello and Chris Whelen on testing restrictions. Mar. 2-3, 2020.

Personal correspondence (e-mail) with Erlaine Bello on isolation procedures, Mar. 5, 2020.

"Physicians work out treatment guideline for coronavirus." *Korea Biomedical Review*, Feb. 13, 2020.

Mahalaxmi Iyer et al. "COVID-19: an update on diagnostic and therapeutic approaches." *BMB Reports* 53, no. 4 (2020): 191–205.

Terry Gross. "Dr. Anthony Fauci." *Fresh Air* (podcast), National Public Radio, Feb. 4, 2021.

Sam Adler-Bell. "Doctor Do-Little: The Case Against Anthony Fauci." *The Drift*, Jan 24, 2021.

"Hawai'i Department of Health Prepares For 2019 Novel Coronavirus." Department of Health, Jan. 29, 2020.

"Hawai'i Department of Health Notified of Confirmed COVID-19 Case Who Traveled to Maui and Oahu." Department of Health, Feb. 14, 2020.

Colleen Uechi and Lee Imada. "Japanese visitor with coronavirus visited Maui." *Maui News*, Feb. 15, 2020.

Kristen Consillio. "Lack of protective gear, erratic policies leave Maui hospital staff fearful of coronavirus infection." *Honolulu Star-Advertiser*, Apr. 11, 2020.

Kristen Consillio. "Maui Memorial Medical Center declares COVID-19 outbreak 'closed.'" *Honolulu Star-Advertiser*, May 20, 2020.

Kristen Consillio. "Hawaii's first case of coronavirus confirmed, Gov. David Ige announces." *Honolulu Star-Advertiser*, Mar. 6, 2020.

"Hawaii Updates: What We're Learning About Coronavirus Today." Hawaii Public Radio, Mar. 9, 2020.

"Hawai'i Department of Health Issues Spring Break Guidelines For Families To Take Action Against COVID-19." Department of Health, Mar. 13, 2020.

"COVID-19: March 16 update from UH president." University of Hawai'i News, Mar. 16, 2020.

"Hawai'i Department of Health Announces 3rd COVID-19 Death." Department of Health, Apr. 3, 2020.

Robbie Dingeman. "Tracking Coronavirus in Hawai'i." *Honolulu*, Mar. 18, 2020.

"Nighttime curfew to go into effect starting Friday, March 20 in support of emergency efforts." County of Kauai, Mar. 18, 2020.

Personal correspondence (e-mail) with Scott Gallacher on PPE, hydroxychloroquine, and COVID-19 research, Mar. 22, 2020.

Chapter Four

Cathie Anderson and Darrell Smith. "Coronavirus patient at UC Davis Medical Center since Feb. 19 wasn't tested for days." *Sacramento Bee*, Feb. 26, 2020.

Roni Rabin. "C.D.C. Confirms First Possible Community Transmission of Coronavirus in U.S.," *New York Times*, Feb. 26, 2020.

"Tracking a pandemic: Q&A with a COVID-19 detective." Fred Hutch News, Mar. 13, 2020.

Trevor Bedford (@trvrb). "I posted back in Feb 8 with this simple model . . ." Twitter, Mar. 13, 2020, 6:49 p.m.

Mary Hudetz et al. "Nursing homes in Washington state struggled with adequate staffing for years. Then coronavirus struck." *Seattle Times*, Sep. 27, 2020.

Ken Budd. "Where is all the PPE?" Association of American Medical Colleges, Mar. 27, 2020.

Martha Blum (@Chenbariatrics1). "Notes from the front lines . . ." Twitter, Mar. 8, 2020, 7:39 a.m.

Caitlyn Stulpin. "First reports of COVID-19 in New York were preceded by uptick in ILI." Healio, Jun. 9, 2020.

"New York State Department of Health 2019–2020 Flu Monitoring Archives" page, New York State website.

Emily Czachor. "Resurfaced Tweets Show New York and San Francisco Mayors' Strikingly Different Coronavirus Messages on Same Day One Month Ago." *Newsweek*, Apr 6, 2020.

Paul Sax. "COVID-19's Siege on Elmhurst Hospital in New York City—An Interview with Dr. Eric Bressman." *Open Forum Infectious Diseases* 7, no. 6 (2020).

Noah Higgins Dunn et al. "New York officials confirm second case of coronavirus in state, identify case as community spread." CNBC, Mar. 3, 2020.

Chris Francescani. "Timeline: The first 100 days of New York Gov. Andrew Cuomo's COVID-19 response." ABC News, Jun. 17, 2020.

Jessica Glenza et al. "'It's what was happening in Italy': the hospital at the center of New York's Covid-19 crisis." *The Guardian*, Mar. 27, 2020.

Joe Ruiz. "Cuomo says New York followed federal guidelines when sending coronavirus patients to nursing homes." CNN, May 24, 2020.

Marina Villeneuve and Jennifer Peltz. "NY count: 6,300 virus patients were sent to nursing homes." *Washington Post*, Jul. 6, 2020.

Tracey Tully. "After Anonymous Tip, 17 Bodies Found at Nursing Home Hit by Virus." *New York Times*, Apr. 17, 2020.

Carl Campanile and Nolan Hicks. "Democrats slam 'lying' Andrew Cuomo over COVID-19 nursing home scandal." *New York Post*, Feb. 15, 2021.

Michael Goodwin. "Gov. Cuomo's 'heartless' distortions can't hide the truth: Goodwin." *New York Post*, Feb. 15, 2021.

Paul LeBlanc. "New York Gov. Andrew Cuomo's Covid-19 controversy, explained." CNN, Feb. 15, 2021.

Guidance for Infection Control and Prevention of Coronavirus Disease 2019 (COVID-19) in Nursing Homes. Centers for Medicare and Medicaid Services, Mar. 13, 2020.

David Rutz. "Celebrity salute to Andrew Cuomo at Emmy ceremony draws mockery: 'How embarrassing.'" Fox News, Feb. 16, 2021.

Erik Wemple. "Opinion: CNN's Chris Cuomo is reminding us why conflicts of interest poison the news." *Washington Post*, Feb. 16, 2021.

MJ Lee and Mark Morales. "Cuomo said 'he can destroy me': NY assemblyman alleges governor threatened him over nursing homes scandal." CNN, Feb 17, 2021.

Marc Thiessen. "Opinion: Cuomo hid covid-19 data. But it was worse than just a coverup." *Washington Post*, Feb. 17, 2021.

Griff Witte. "South Dakota's governor resisted ordering people to stay home. Now it has one of the nation's largest coronavirus hot spots." Washington Post, Apr. 13, 2020.

Chapter Five

"New COVID-19 forecasts: US hospitals could be overwhelmed by the second week of April by demand for ICU beds, and US deaths could total 81,000 by July." Institute for Health Metrics & Evaluation (IHME), Mar. 26, 2020.

Neil Ferguson et al. *Report 9: Impact of non-pharmaceutical interventions (NPIs) to reduce COVID-19 mortality and healthcare demand.* Imperial College COVID-19 Response Team, Mar. 16, 2020.

COVID-19 Hospital Impact Model for Epidemics (CHIME).

University of Pennsylvania.

Personal correspondence (e-mail) with Chris Whelen and Erlaine Bello on testing restrictions, Feb. 29–Mar. 2, 2020.

Personal correspondence (e-mail) with Chris Whelen, Nogi Masayugi, Erlaine Bello, and James Joyner, Apr. 8–9, 2020.

Personal correspondence (e-mail) with David Derauf, Apr. 25–26, 2020.

Personal correspondence (e-mail) with Eric Crawley, Mar. 26–27, 2020.

Personal correspondence (e-mail) with Jerry Murphy on effectiveness of HI-EMA response, May 6, 2021.

Václav Havel. *Open Letters: Selected Writings 1965–1990* Vintage Books, 1992.

"UH medical school professor plays key role in state's COVID-19 response." University of Hawaiʻi News, May 4, 2020.

Annalisa Burgos. "Hawaii ramps up COVID-19 crisis response with new pandemic unit." KITV4, Sep. 12, 2020.

Peter Goodman. "Sweden Has Become the World's Cautionary Tale." *New York Times*, Jul. 7, 2020.

John Barry. "A Warning to the United States From the Author of 'The Great Influenza.'" New York Times, Aug. 18, 2020.

Paul Brewbaker. Hawaiʻi resident consumer spending plummeted prior to stay-at-home order. Source data from Opportunity Insights, Affinity Solutions, and Hawaiʻi Data Collaborative.

Ryan Tsuji and Yunji de Nies. "VIDEO: Economist Paul Brewbaker discusses Hawaii's outlook on the Star-Advertiser's Spotlight Hawaii." *Star-Advertiser*, Aug. 5, 2020.

Michael Smithson. "Data from 45 countries show containing COVID vs saving the economy is a false dichotomy." The Conversation, Nov. 25, 2020.

"The Zero Covid strategy protects people and economies more effectively." Institut Économique Molinari, Apr. 10, 2021.

Miquel Oliu-Barton et al. "SARS-CoV-2 elimination, not mitigation, creates best outcomes for health, the economy, and civil liberties." *The Lancet*, Apr. 28, 2021.

Michael Mina (@michaelmina_lab). "On TTI as a control measure: . . ." Twitter, Feb. 17, 2021, 5:06 p.m.

Martin Kulldorff, Sunetra Gupta, and Jay Bhattacharya. "The Great Barrington Declaration." Petition, Great Barrington, Massachusetts, 2020.

David Gorski. "The Great Barrington Declaration: COVID-19 deniers follow the path laid down by creationists, HIV/AIDS denialists, and climate science deniers." Science-Based Medicine, Oct. 12, 2020.

Nisreen Alwan et al. "Scientific consensus on the COVID-19 pandemic: we need to act now." *The Lancet*, Oct. 31, 2020.

Nisreen Alwan et al. "The Jon Snow Memorandum." Petition, 2020.

Chapter Six

John Barry. *The Great Influenza: The Epic Story of the Deadliest Plague in History*. Penguin Books, 2004.

Phil Stewart and Idrees Ali. "Coronavirus clue? Most cases aboard U.S. aircraft carrier are symptom-free." Reuters, Apr. 16, 2020.

The RECOVERY Collaborative Group. "Effect of Hydroxychloroquine in Hospitalized Patients with Covid-19." *New England Journal of*

Medicine 383 (2020): 2030–2040.

Christi Young. "A COVID-19 Timeline: How Honolulu Got To This Pont." *Honolulu*, Mar.5, 2021.

Christina O'Connor. "Nearly 200 people arrested for violating Hawaii's 14-day mandatory quarantine." *Pacific Business News*, Jul. 17, 2020.

Personal correspondence with Erlaine Bello, Mar. 27, 2020.

Personal correspondence with Heath Chung, Apr. 2, 2020.

Chapter Seven

Bruce Soll. Reflections & Recommendations. May, 2020.

Roger Seheult (MedCram - Medical Lectures Explained CLEARLY). "Vitamin D and COVID 19: The Evidence for Prevention and Treatment of Coronavirus (SARS CoV 2)." YouTube video, 1:00:23, Dec. 10, 2020.

Siddhartha Mukherjee. "Why Does The Pandemic Seem To Be Hitting Some Countries Harder Than Others?" *The New Yorker*, Feb. 22, 2021.

Jose Maria Leon Cabrera and Anatoly Kurmanaev. "As Bodies Accumulate, So Do Fears of a High Coronavirus Toll in Ecuador." *New York Times*, Apr. 14, 2020.

Anita Hofschneider. "10 Family Members, 4 Bedrooms And 'A Dream To Have Your Own Place.'" Civil Beat, Nov .15, 2018.

"Civil Beat-HNN poll: Despite partisan divide, support for COVID-19 orders is broad." Hawai'i News Now, May 27, 2020.

Howard Koh. "We need one response—not 50—to fight Covid-19." STAT, May 22, 2020.

Libby Cathey. "Trump now calling coronavirus fight a 'war' with an 'invisible enemy.'" ABC News, Mar. 17, 2020.

Amber Phillips. "Was the stock market the object of Trump's 'don't create a panic' coronavirus approach?" *Washington Post*, Sep. 10, 2020.

Donald Trump. Remarks by President Trump on the Jobs Numbers Report. Jul. 2, 2020.

Jonathan Lemire, Jill Colvin, and Alan Suderman. "Amid protests, Trump talks of war—and reelection." AP News, Jun. 1, 2020.

Ed Yong. "How the Pandemic Defeated America." *The Atlantic*, Aug. 4, 2020.

Drew Altman. "Understanding the US failure on coronavirus—an essay by Drew Altman." *British Medical Journal* 370 (2020).

Cameron Peters. "A detailed timeline of all the ways Trump failed to respond to the coronavirus." Vox, Jun. 8, 2020.

Chris Riotta. "Rand Paul defends himself over failure to self-isolate as he's slammed for 'violating doctor's oath.'" *The Independent*, Mar. 23, 2020.

Aaron Blake. "'We just need some more optimism': Rand Paul's crusade against Anthony Fauci takes a curious turn." *Washington Post*, Jun. 30, 2020.

Jeremy Chisenhall. "Rand Paul bashes his 'Twitter haters,' touts natural immunity over COVID vaccine." *Lexington Herald Leader*, Nov. 18, 2020.

Dominick Mastrangelo. "Rand Paul says Fauci owes parents and students an apology over pandemic measures." *The Hill*, Nov. 30, 2020.

Morgan Gstalter. "Rand Paul says COVID-19 survivors should 'throw away their masks, go to restaurants, live again.'" *The Hill*, Nov. 13, 2020.

Aaron Blake. "'Here we go again with the theater': Fauci pushes back on Rand Paul's amateur epidemiology—again." *Washington Post*, Mar. 18, 2021.

Hannah Kuchler and Andrew Edgecliffe-Johnson. "How New York's missteps let Covid-19 overwhelm the US." *Financial Times*, Oct. 21, 2020.

John Stossel. "Hypocritical Politicians Violate Their Own Coronavirus Restrictions." Reason, Jan. 27, 2021.

Teo Armus. "California Democrats urged people to stay home—and then did the opposite at restaurants and holiday parties." *Washington Post*, Dec. 2, 2020.

Ted Barrett. "Pelosi's office acknowledges indoor hair appointment, violating San Francisco Covid-19 restrictions." CNN, Sep. 2, 2020.

Maanvi Singh. "How California went from a leader in the Covid fight to a state in despair." *The Guardian*, Dec. 29, 2020.

"Governor Gavin Newsom Issues Stay at Home Order." The website of the Office of Governor Gavin Newsom, Mar. 19, 2020.

"California Health Officials Announce a Regional Stay at Home Order Triggered by ICU Capacity." The website of the Office of Governor Gavin Newsom, Dec. 3, 2020.

Neil Gong. "California gave people the 'right' to be homeless—but little help finding homes." *Washington Post*, May 20, 2021.

"A Timeline of COVID-19 Developments in 2020." *American Journal of Managed Care* website, Jan. 1, 2021.

Kristen Holmes, Nick Valencia, and Curt Devine. "CDC woes bring Director Redfield's troubled past as an AIDS researcher to light." CNN, Jun. 5, 2020.

Valerie Strauss. "Democratic lawmakers probing whether CDC guidelines on reopening schools were influenced by political pressure." *Washington Post*, Jul. 28, 2020.

Lena Sun. "CDC reverses controversial coronavirus guidelines for testing people without symptoms." *Washington Post*, Sep. 18, 2020.

Johns Hopkins University. "Understanding Changing Guidance on Mask Use." Hub, Apr. 24, 2020.

Grace Panetta. "Fauci says he doesn't regret telling Americans not to wear masks at the beginning of the pandemic." Business Insider, Jul. 16, 2020.

Zeynep Tufekci. "Why Telling People They Don't Need Masks Backfired." *New York Times*, Mar. 17, 2020.

Kate Murphy. "UNC professor challenged top health officials about COVID-19 guidance. She was right." *The News & Observer*, Jan. 29, 2021.

Katherine Randall et al. "How Did We Get Here: What Are Droplets and Aerosols and How Far Do They Go? A Historical Perspective on the Transmission of Respiratory Infectious Diseases." Social Science Research Network, Apr. 28, 2021.

Eran Bendavid et al. "COVID-19 Antibody Seroprevalence in Santa Clara County, California." medRxiv, Apr. 17, 2020.

Gideon Meyerowitz-Katz. "A systematic review and meta-analysis of published research data on COVID-19 infection fatality rates." *International Journal of Infectious Diseases* 101 (2020): 138–148.

Lauren Bauer et al. "Ten facts about COVID-19 and the U.S. economy." Brookings, Sep. 17, 2020.

Erica Chenoweth and Jeremy Pressman. "This summer's Black Lives Matter protesters were overwhelmingly peaceful, our research finds."

Washington Post, Oct. 16, 2020.

Brendan Kiley et al. “Seattle police clear CHOP protest zone.” *Seattle Times*, Jul. 1, 2020.

“Open letter advocating for an anti-racist public health response to demonstrations against systemic injustice occurring during the COVID-19 pandemic.” Petition, 2020.

“Over 1,000 health experts sign letter supporting anti-Black racism protests despite COVID-19 risks.” CBC Radio, Jun. 8, 2020.

Julia Marcus and Gregg Gonsalves. “Public-Health Experts Are Not Hypocrites.” *The Atlantic*, Jun. 11, 2020.

Jason Lemon. “Chair of Congressional Black Caucus Says She Does Not Think Defunding Police Is ‘the Appropriate Thing to Do.’” *Newsweek*, Jun. 9, 2020.

“James Clyburn: ‘defund the police’ slogan may have hurt Democrats at polls.” *The Guardian*, Nov. 8, 2020.

“As violence surges, some question Portland axing police unit.” Associated Press, Mar. 6, 2021.

Sam Harris. “Can We Pull Back From The Brink?” *Making Sense* (podcast) transcript, Jun. 18, 2020.

Saturday Night Live. “Dr. Anthony Fauci Cold Open - SNL.” YouTube video, 3:12, Apr. 25, 2020.

Seth Cohen. “Is Fauci a ‘Deep State’ Doctor? The Conspiracy Theory That Is Sickening America.” *Forbes*, Jul. 14, 2020.

Michael Gerson. “Opinion: Why tearing down Fauci is essential to the MAGA myth.” Washington Post, Apr. 5, 2021.

Adrianna Rodriguez. "2020 wasn't 'just a random bad year,' health experts say: COVID-19 made it one of the deadliest in US history." *USA Today*, Jan. 21, 2021.

Chapter Eight

"COVID-19 Information Hub" page, Hawai'i Emergency Management Agency website.

"Proclamations, Orders, and Rules re:COVID-19" page, City and County of Honolulu website.

Centers for Disease Control and Prevention. "CDC calls on Americans to wear masks to prevent COVID-19 spread." CDC Newsroom, Jul. 14, 2020.

Catherine Marfin. "Why did the recommendation on wearing face masks change? Curious Texas investigates." *Dallas Morning News*, Apr. 8, 2020.

Megan Molteni. "The 60-Year-Old Scientific Screwup That Helped Covid Kill." *Wired*, May 13, 2021.

Brian Krans. "25% of People Believe Unproven Conspiracy Theories About COVID-19." Healthline, Jun. 12, 2020.

Brittany Lyte. "Inside Hawaii's Ambitious Mobile Virus-Testing Operation." Civil Beat, Apr. 27, 2020.

Personal correspondence (e-mail) with David Derauf, Chad Meyer, and Chad Taniguchi, Aug. 4, 2020.
Notes on mayor's meeting (documented in same e-mail), Jul. 30, 2020.

Personal correspondence (e-mail) with David Derauf and Jerry Murphy, Apr. 17–18, 2020.

Nicole Tame. "Bars on Oahu allowed to re-open under COVID-19 guidelines." KITV4, Jun. 19, 2020.

"Hawaii Updates: 41 New COVID Cases Set Record; Bar, Gym Clusters May Prompt Reopening Rollback." Hawaii Public Radio, Jul. 7, 2020.

Corrado Rizzi. "Hawaii Governor, Honolulu Mayor Facing Class Action Over COVID-19 Shutdown Orders for Bar, Nightlife Industry." Class Action Newswire, Oct. 20, 2020.

Jason Beaubien. "Singapore Was A Shining Star In COVID-19 Control—Until It Wasn't." National Public Radio, May 3, 2020.

Brendan Saloner, Kalind Parish, Julie Ward, et al. "COVID-19 Cases and Deaths in Federal and State Prisons." *Journal of the American Medical Association* 324, no. 6 (2020) 602–603.

Chapter Nine

Michael Mina, Roy Parker, and Daniel Larremore. "Rethinking COVID-19 Test Sensitivity—A Strategy for Containment." *New England Journal of Medicine* 383, no. 120 (2020).

Trevor Bedford (@trvrb). "This is the Apollo program of our times." Twitter, Mar. 18, 2020, 6:07 p.m.

Stephen Hahn and Jeffrey Shuren. "Coronavirus (COVID-19) Update: FDA Authorizes First Antigen Test to Help in the Rapid Detection of the Virus that Causes COVID-19 in Patients." FDA, May 9, 2020.

Jessica Prince-Guerra et al. "Evaluation of Abbott BinaxNOW Rapid Antigen Tests for SARS-CoV-2 Infection at Two Community-Based Testing Sites—Pima County, Arizona, November 3–17, 2020)." *Morbidity and Mortality Weekly Report* 70, no. 3 (2021): 100–105.

William Lanier et al. "COVID-19 Testing to Sustain In-Person

Instruction and Extracurricular Activities in High Schools—Utah, November 2020–March 2021." *Morbidity and Mortality Weekly Report* 70, no. 21 (2021): 785–791.

Tim Mercer and Marc Salit. "Testing at scale during the COVID-19 pandemic." *Nature Reviews Genetics* 22 (2021): 415–426.

Patrick Sullivan. *Intellectual Anarchy: The Art of Disruptive Innovation.* Oceanit, 2020.

Notes from telephone interview with Patrick Sullivan, Feb. 24, 2021.

Notes from telephone interview with David Watumull, Mar. 6, 2021.

Mahealani Richardson. "Hawai'i company in mad dash to secure emergency authorization for COVID-19 saliva test." Hawaii News Now, Dec. 25, 2020.

Eleni Avedaño. "Growing Use of Rapid Testing Provides A 'Degree Of Safety' As Hawaii Reopens." Civil Beat, Jun. 4, 2021.

Jerry Murphy et al. Letter from healthcare professionals to Governor David Ige, May 4, 2020.

Lynn Kawano. "More volunteers sought for state's new contact tracing program." Hawaii News Now, Jun. 2, 2020.

"UH begins training COVID-19 contact tracers." University of Hawai'i News, Jun. 7, 2020.

Personal correspondence with City and County of Honolulu medical advisory group, Jun. 11, 2020.

Jonathan Dworkin, David Derauf, Tim Brown, Chad Meyer, Sumner La Croix. "I Maluhia Kakou: A Plan For Opening Hawaii Safely." Civil Beat, Jun. 11, 2020.

Tim Brown, Sumner La Croix, and F. DeWolfe Miller. Prevention of Travel-Related Reintroduction of COVID-19 Infection in the State of Hawaii. UHERO, Jun. 9, 2020.

Catherine Cruz. "Petition Raises Concerns Over Transparency and Meaningful Testing." [Interview with Jonathan Dworkin and David Ige.] *The Conversation* (podcast), Hawaii Public Radio, Jun. 8, 2020.

Chapter Ten

Jason Horowitz. "The Lost Days That Made Bergamo a Coronavirus Tragedy." *New York Times*, Nov. 29, 2020.

Melissa Hawkins. "The US isn't in a second wave of coronavirus—the first wave never ended." The Conversation, Jun. 30, 2020.

Michael Martina and Ben Klayman. "Michigan Governor Whitmer faces mainstream backlash against shutdown." Reuters, May 20, 2020.

Dan Sewell and Andrew Welsh-Huggins. "Ohio Gov. Mike DeWine's conflicting COVID-19 tests raise backlash." *Cincinnati Enquirer*, Aug. 9, 2020.

Emily Stewart. "Anti-maskers explain themselves." Vox, Aug. 7, 2020.

Cleve Wootson et al. "Coronavirus ravaged Florida, as Ron DeSantis sidelined scientists and followed Trump." *Washington Post*, Jul. 25, 2020.

Griff Witte and Rachel Weiner. "Sun Belt hospitals are feeling the strain from virus' surge—and bracing for worse." *Washington Post*, Jul. 16, 2020.

Sarah Crump and MaryAnn Placheril. "The Sun Belt's COVID-19 surge stalls economic recovery in the region." Brookings, Aug. 14, 2020.

Apoorva Mandavilli. "C.D.C. Testing Guidance Was Published Against

Scientist's Objections." *New York Times*, Sep. 17, 2020.

Ashley Mizuo. "Failure to Communicate: State Provides Inadequate COVID-19 Outreach, Services To Pacific Islanders." Hawaii Public Radio, Sep. 3, 2020.

DeWolfe Miller et al. "Unique pattern of COVID-19 infection in the State of Hawaiʻi." *International Journal of Infectious Diseases* 103 (2021): 298–299.

"3 COVID-19 deaths on Oahu as Hawaiʻi sees 310 new coronavirus cases and 12 hospitalizations." *Honolulu Star-Advertiser*, Aug. 29, 2020.

Twelfth Proclamation Related To The COVID-19 Emergency. "Emergency Proclamations" page, website of the Governor of the State of Hawaiʻi David Y. Ige, Aug. 20, 2020.

Caleb Jones. "Hawaii visitor arrivals down almost 98% in July as coronavirus pandemic decimates tourism." *USA Today*, Aug. 28, 2020.

Kapono Chong-Hanssen and JoAnn Yukimura. "Hawaiʻi as a kipuka: a COVID-free state where we can thrive." *The Garden Island*, Sep. 6, 2020.

Notes on meeting with Governor David Ige, Aug. 4, 2020.

"Proclamations, Orders, and Rules re:COVID-19" page, City and County of Honolulu website.

Ani Nalbandian et al. "Post-acute COVID-19 syndrome." *Nature Medicine* 27 (2021): 601–615.

Zubin Damania (ZDoggMD). "Here's What Masks ACTUALLY Do." Facebook video, 4:38, Aug. 18, 2020.

Nikki Schenfeld. "HPD issues hundreds of citations on first day of beach closure." KHON2, Aug. 8, 2020.

"Protesters rally in opposition of stay-at-home orders, other COVID-19 response efforts." Hawaii News Now, Sep. 7, 2020.

Christina Jedra and Yoohyun Jung. "Easy Targets? Some O'ahu Homeless Have Been Ticketed Dozens Of Times During The Pandemic." Civil Beat, Nov. 2, 2020.

Christina Jedra. "Honolulu Taxpayers Will Foot The Bill For HPD Overtime Abuse." Civil Beat, Dec. 3, 2020.

Christina Jedra. "What Did HPD Do To Prevent Another Kealoha Scandal? Not Much, Chief Says." Civil Beat, Dec. 16, 2020.

Christina Jedra. "Feds Examining Honolulu Police CARES Spending on ATVs, Robot Dog." Civil Beat, Mar. 9, 2021.

Notes on conversation with Josh Stanbro, Apr. 5, 2021.

Notes on conversation with Kirk Caldwell, Jul. 15, 2021.

"Mayor Kirk Caldwell's Foolish Plan To Fatten HPD With CARES Money." Civil Beat, Sep. 22, 2020.

Rosemarie Barnardo. "U.S. Surgeon General Jerome Adams to be arraigned for beach park closure violation." *Honolulu Star-Advertiser*, Oct. 22, 2020.

Noah Feldman. "The Big Data Revolution." Deep Background with Noah Feldman (podcast), Pushkin, Dec. 2, 2020.

John Beigel et al for the ACCT-1 Study Group Members. "Remdesivir for the Treatment of COVID-19—Final Report." *New England Journal of Medicine* 383 (2020): 1813–1826.

The RECOVERY Collaborative Group. Dexamethasone in Hospitalized Patients with COVID-19. *New England Journal of Medicine*, Feb. 25, 2021.

WHO Solidarity Trial Consortium. "Repurposed Antiviral Drugs for COVID-19—Interim WHO Solidarity Trial Results." *New England Journal of Medicine*, Feb. 11, 2021.

Ventura Simonovich et al for the PlasmAr Study Group. "A Randomized Trial of Convalescent Plasma in COVID-19 Severe Pneumonia." *New England Journal of Medicine*, Fen. 18, 2021.

"Coronavirus (COVID-19) Update: FDA Authorizes Monoclonal Antibody [Bamlanivimab] for Treatment of COVID-19." FDA, Nov. 9, 2020.

"Coronavirus (COVID-19) Update: FDA Authorizes Monoclonal Antibodies [Casirivimab and Imdevimab] for COVID-19." FDA, Nov. 21, 2020.

Chapter Eleven

Personal correspondence with Ryan Honda and Libby Char, Aug. 20, 2020.

Timothy Hurley. "Mayor Kirk Caldwell announces new stay-at-home, work-from-home order for Oahu." *Honolulu Star-Advertiser*, Aug. 25, 2020.

Ani Nalbandian. "Post-acute COVID-19 syndrome." *Nature Medicine* 27 (2021): 601–615.

Personal correspondence with David Derauf and Chad Meyers, Aug. 4, 2020.

Personal correspondence with Tim Brown, Aug. 9, 2020.

Sarah Park's letter to the Senate Special Committee on COVID-19, "Re: Contact Tracing," Jul. 29, 2020.

Senate Special Committee on COVID-19, Informational Briefing on Aug. 6, 2020.

Yoohyun Jung. "State Officials Are Overusing Privacy Excuse To Withhold COVID-19 Data." Civil Beat, Sep. 4, 2020.

Allison Schaefers. "HGEA grievance cites just 15 contact tracers on Oahu, where COVID-19 cases are surging." *Honolulu Star-Advertiser*, Aug. 10, 2020.

Mark Carpenter. "'Out of Control': Union grievance filed against DOH as criticism of pandemic response builds." Hawaii News Now, Aug. 11, 2020.

Stewart Yerton. "Hawaii's Contact Tracing Effort Falls Short of National Standards." Civil Beat, Aug. 12, 2020.

Stewart Yerton. "This Whistleblower Exposed The Health Department's COVID-19 Shortcomings." Civil Beat, Aug. 14, 2020.

Mahealani Richardson. "Whistleblower describes a Health Department 'struggling to keep up.'" Hawaii News Now, Aug. 14, 2020.

Stewart Yerton. "California Congresswoman Wants Answers On Hawaii's Virus Response Effort." Civil Beat, Aug. 19, 2020.

Notes on conversation with anonymous, Apr. 8, 2021.

Allison Schaefers. "Gov. David Ige defends Hawaii's contact tracing." *Honolulu Star-Advertiser*, Aug. 20, 2020.

Audrey McAvoy. "Emails show strain on Hawaii administration amid coronavirus pandemic." Honolulu Star-Advertiser, Jun. 5, 2021.

Kevin Dayton. "Anderson, Espinda Out In Ige Cabinet Shake-Up." Civil Beat, Aug 31, 2020.

Allison Schaefers and Mark Ladao. "Embattled state epidemiologist Dr. Sarah Park put on paid leave." *Honolulu Star-Advertiser*, Sep. 4, 2020.

"Hawaii governor criticizes senators over health inspection." Associated Press, Aug. 17, 2020.

Chad Blair. "Chad Blair: David Ige, The Governor Who Cannot Govern." Civil Beat, May 19, 2020.

Chad Blair. "Chad Blair: Can David Ige Be Impeached?" Civil Beat, Sep. 3, 2020.

Personal correspondence with Elizabeth Char, Aug. 31, 2020.

Allison Schaefers. "State Health Director Bruce Anderson and Public Safety Department Director Nolan Espinda are leaving their posts." *Honolulu Star-Advertiser*, Sep. 1, 2020.

Chapter Twelve

"Covid: US death toll passes 200,000." BBC News, Sep. 23, 2020.

JP Keenan and Ivan Pereira. "For many white evangelicals, the Supreme Court makeup solidifies their support for President Trump." ABC News, Oct. 16, 2020.

Olga Khazan. "A Failure of Empathy Led to 200,000 Deaths. It Has Deep Roots." *The Atlantic*, Sep. 22, 2020.

Grace Dean and Andrew Dunn. "Donald Trump and his son Donald Trump Jr., without evidence, accuse Pfizer of deliberately waiting until after Election Day to release its COVID-19 vaccine trial results." *Business Insider*, Nov. 10, 2020.

Thomas Sowell. *Black Rednecks and White Liberals*. Encounter Books, 2005.

Personal correspondence with Libby Char, David Derauf, and Hiro Toiya, Sep. 6, 2020.

Keun-Sang Kwon et al. "Evidence of Long-Distance Droplet Transmission of SARS-CoV-2 by Direct Air Flow in a Restaurant in Korea." *Journal of Korean Medical Science* 35, no. 46 (2020).

Gerry Guy et al. "Association of State-Issued Mask Mandates and Allowing On-Premises Restaurant Dining with County-Level COVID-19 Case and Death Growth Rates—United States, March 1–December 31, 2020." *Morbidity and Mortality Weekly Report* 70, no. 10 (2021): 350–354.

Jess Millar et al. "Risk factors for increased COVID-19 case-fatality in the United States: A county-level analysis during the first wave." medRxiv, Feb. 24, 2021.

Jan Brauner et al. "Inferring the effectiveness of government interventions against COVID-19." *Science*, Feb. 19, 2021.

Serina Chang et al. "Mobility network models of COVID-19 explain inequities and inform reopening." Nature 589 (2020): 82–87.

Neil Paine. "Experts Think The Economy Would Be Stronger If COVID-19 Lockdowns Had Been More Aggressive." FiveThirtyEight, Sep. 22, 2020.

"Reopening Strategy (Honolulu's Tier System" page, One Oahu website.

Personal correspondence with Tim Brown, Sep. 26, 2020.

Darragh O'Carroll. "How Hawaii Can Get Coronavirus Right In Twelve Steps." *Darragh O'Carroll M.D.* (Medium blog), Nov. 23, 2020.

Kapono Chong-Hannsen et al. "Kaua'i County Council and schools reopening." *The Garden Island*, Feb. 23, 2021.

Presentation on Department of Education Strategies for Safe Reopening of Elementary and Secondary Schools to More In-Person Learning for Fourth Quarter of 2020–2021 School Year. Department of Education, Mar. 4, 2021.

Suevon Lee. "DOE Doesn't Expect Schools To Fully Reopen Until Next Year." Civil Beat, Mar. 15, 2021.

Personal correspondence with Chad Taniguchi, Nov. 5, 2020.
"Covid19 coronavirus: Tahiti pandemic death toll now 26, with cases over 6400." *New Zealand Herald*, Oct. 26, 2020.

Personal correspondence with David Derauf, Jun. 13, 2020.

Personal correspondence with DeWolfe Miller, Jul. 7, 2020.

Personal correspondence with David Derauf, Jul. 4, 2020.

Personal correspondence with Darragh O'Carroll, Oct. 2, 2020.

Steve O'Neal. "Without Data And Stress-Tested Protocols, It's Foolish To Reopen Hawaii." Civil Beat, Oct. 2, 2020.

Suevon Lee. "Can Hawaii Bring Students Back To The Classroom Safely Yet?" Civil Beat, Nov. 6, 2020.

Mel Rapoza. "Dr. Jonathan Dworkin and David Derauf have a no-fluff Covid-19 discussion – December 9, 2020." YouTube video, 1:30:03, Dec. 9, 2020.

Notes from City and County of Honolulu Medical Advisory Committee meeting on Oct. 8, 2020. Hotel room data shared by Victoria Fan.

Personal correspondence with David Derauf, Sep. 10, 2020.

Kevin Dayton. "Hilo Veterans Home Deaths: Rev. Richard Uejo Ministered To Many In Hawaii." Civil Beat, Sep. 18, 2020.

Stephanie Salmons. "Kim to Ige: Remove Avalon as veterans home manager." *Hawaii Tribune Herald*, Sep. 21, 2020.

"Avalon Health Care replaced as managing company of Yukio Okutsu State Veterans Home." KHON2, Sep. 25, 2020.

Personal correspondence with Darragh O'Carroll, Sep. 27, 2020.
Pacific Islander cluster response meeting with Mayor Harry Kim, Oct 20, 2020.

Rosemarie Bernardo. "Harry Kim ends third terms as 'voice of authority.'" *Honolulu Star-Advertiser*, Dec. 7, 2020.

Eleni Avendaño. "Hawaii Grapples With How To Use Stockpile Of Rapid COVID-19 Tests." Civil Beat, Feb. 23, 2021.

Eleni Avendaño. "Hawaii Wants To Give Away COVID-19 Tests, But Not For Big Island Airport Screening." Civil Beat, Mar. 2, 2021.

Eleni Avendaño. "Vaccines Open To 16 And Up On Kauai And Big Island." Civil Beat, Apr. 2, 2021.

Chapter Thirteen

Sandy Cohen. "The fastest vaccine in history." UCLA Health, Dec. 10, 2020.

Cuiling Zhang et al. "Advances in mRNA Vaccines for Infectious Diseases." *Frontiers in Immunology* 10 (2019): 594.

Ian Tizard. "Vaccination against coronaviruses in domestic animals." *Vaccine* 38, no. 33 (2020): 5123–1530.

Jennifer Dan et al. "Immunological memory to SARS-CoV-2 assessed for greater than six months after infection." bioRxiv, Dec. 18, 2020.

Eric Lau et al. "Neutralizing antibody titers in SARS-CoV-2 infections." *Nature Communications* 12 (2021).

Christian Gaebler et al. "Evolution of antibody immunity to SARS-CoV-2." *Nature* 591 (2021): 639–644.

Jonathan Yewdell. "Individuals cannot rely on COVID-19 herd immunity: Durable immunity to viral disease is limited to viruses with obligate viremic spread." *PLOS Pathogens* 17, no. 4 (2021).

Pfizer-BioNTech COVID-19 Vaccine. FDA briefing document, Dec. 10, 2020.

Moderna COVID-19 Vaccine. FDA briefing document, Dec. 17, 2020.

Janssen Ad26.Cov2.S Vaccine for the Prevention of COVID-19. FDA briefing document, Feb. 26, 2021.

Noah Feldman. "What We Know About the COVID-19 Vaccines." *Deep Background with Noah Feldman* (podcast), Pushkin, Nov. 17, 2020.

Kyle Allred (MedCram – Medical Lectures Explained CLEARLY). "COVID 19 Vaccine Deep Dive: Safety, Immunity, RNA Production, (Pfizer Vaccine / Moderna Vaccine)." YouTube video, 34:28, Dec. 16, 2020.

Lisa Jackson et al for the mRNA-1273 Study Group [Moderna). "An mRNA Vaccine against SARS-CoV-2—Preliminary Report." *New England Journal of Medicine* 383 (2020): 1920–1931.

Scott Halstead and Leah Katzelnick. "COVID-19 Vaccines: Should We Fear ADE?" *Journal of Infectious Diseases* 222, no. 12 (2020): 1946–1950.

Bert Spector. "The polio vaccine mess holds lessons for the lagging COVID-19 vaccination effort." *Philly Voice*, Jan. 16, 2021.

"What to Do If You Have an Allergic Reaction after Getting a

COVID-19 Vaccine." Centers for Disease Control and Prevention, Mar. 4, 2021.

"Allergic Reactions Including Anaphylaxis After Receipt of the First Dose of Pfizer-BioNTech COVID-19 Vaccine—United States, December 14–23, 2020." *Morbidity and Mortality Weekly Report* 70, no. 2 (2021): 46–51.

Raghavendra Tirupathi et al. "Q&A: What PCPs need to know about COVID-19 vaccines." Healio Primary Care, Jan. 6, 2021.

Janel Miller. "Experts say COVID-19 vaccine should be offered to pregnant women." Healio Primary Care, Jan. 6, 2021.

Laurie McGinley, Carolyn Johnson, Joel Achenbach. "FDA says it 'will rapidly work toward' authorization of Pfizer-BioNTech coronavirus vaccine." *Washington Post*, Dec. 11, 2020.

Christina Maxouris and Jason Hanna. "US Covid-19 hospitalizations at record high for 12th day as FDA says it plans to grant emergency authorization of 2nd vaccine." CNN, Dec. 17, 2020.

Andrew Rambault (arambaut) et al. "Preliminary genomic characterisation of an emergent SARS-CoV-2 lineage in the UK defined by a novel set of spike mutations." Virological, Dec. 8, 2020.

Yang Liu et al. "Neutralizing Activity of BNT162b2-Elicited Serum." *New England Journal of Medicine* 384 (2021): 1466–1468.

Kai Wu et al. "Serum Neutralizing Activity Elicited by mRNA-1273 Vaccine." *New England Journal of Medicine* 384 (2021): 1468–1470.

Colin Pawlowski et al. "FDA-authorized COVID-19 vaccines are effective per real-world evidence synthesized across a multi-state health system." medRxiv, Feb. 18, 2021.

Jocelyn Keehner et al. "SARS-CoV-2 Infection after Vaccination in

Health Care Workers in California." New England Journal of Medicine 384 (2021): 1774–1775.

William Daniel et al. "Early Evidence of the Effect of SARS-CoV-2 Vaccine at One Medical Center." New England Journal of Medicine 384 (2021): 1962–1963.

Mark Thompson et al. "Interim Estimates of Vaccine Effectiveness of BNT162b2 and mRNA-1273 COVID-19 Vaccines in Preventing SARS-CoV-2 Infection Among Health Care Personnel, First Responders, and Other Essential and Frontline Workers—Eight U.S. Locations, December 2020–March 2021." *Morbidity and Mortality Weekly Report* 70, no. 13 (2021): 495–500.

Tamara Pilishvili et al. "Interim Estimates of Vaccine Effectiveness of Pfizer-BioNTech and Moderna COVID-19 Vaccines Among Health Care Personnel—33 U.S. Sites, January–March 2021." *Morbidity and Mortality Weekly Report* 70, no. 20 (2021): 753–758.

Personal correspondence with Tim Brown, Dec. 21, 2020.

New and Emerging Respiratory Virus Threats Advisory Group (NERVTAG) meeting on SARS-CoV-2 variant under investigation, Dec. 18, 2020.

Nicholas Davies et al. "Increased mortality in community-tested cases of SARS-CoV-2 lineage B.1.1.7." *Nature* 593 (2021): 270–274.

Josh Holder, Allison McCann, and Benjamin Mueller. "Rise of Variants in Europe Shows How Dangerous the Virus Can Be." New York Times, Apr. 9, 2021.

Marc Santora and Elian Peltier. "The variant first detected in India is forcing the U.K. to speed up delivery of second doses of vaccine." *New York Times*, May 14, 2021.

Andrew Joseph. "The looming questions scientists need to answer about the new variant of the coronavirus." STAT, Dec. 21, 2020.

Gerard Gallagher. "Pfizer vaccine appears effective against emerging SARS-CoV-2 variants." Healio, Jan. 8, 2021.

"SARS-CoV-2 Variant Classifications and Definitions." Centers for Disease Control and Prevention, Aug. 24, 2021.

Arman Azad. "Coronavirus strains first detected in California are officially 'variants of concern,' CDC says." CNN, Mar. 17, 2021.

Prashant Ranjan et al. "Bioinformatics analysis of SARS-CoV-2 RBD mutant variants and insights into antibody and ACE2 receptor binding." bioRxiv, Apr 3, 2021.

Apoorva Mandavilli. "Vaccines Are Effective Against the New York Variant, Studies Find." *New York Times*, Apr. 22, 2021.

Laith Abu-Raddad et al. "Effectiveness of the BNT162b2 Covid-19 Vaccine against the B.1.1.7 and B.1.351 variants." *New England Journal of Medicine* 385 (2021): 187–189.

Adam Taylor. "Why the world's most vaccinated country is seeing an unprecedented spike in Coronavirus cases." *Washington Post*, May 6, 2021.

Angela Choi et al. "Serum Neutralizing Activity of mRNA-1273 against SARS-CoV-2 Variants." bioRxiv, Jun. 28, 2021.

SARS-CoV-2 variants of concern and variants under investigation in England. Public Health England, Jun. 18, 2021.

Jamie Bernal et al. "Effectiveness of COVID-19 vaccines against the B.1.617.2 variant." medRxiv, May 24, 2021.

Mackenzie Bean and Erica Carbajal. "How vaccines stack up against CDC's 5 variants of concern." *Becker's Hospital Review*, Jun. 20, 2021.

Adam Taylor. "Why the world's most vaccinated country is seeing an unprecedented spike in coronavirus cases." *Washington Post*, May 6, 2021.

Adam Taylor and Paul Schemm. "China's great vaccine hope, Sinopharm, sees reputation darkened amid covid spikes in countries using it." *Washington Post*, Jun. 3, 2021.

Ezgi Hacisuleyman et al. "Vaccine Breakthrough Infections with SARS-CoV-2 Variants." N*ew England Journal of Medicine* 384 (2021): 2212–2218.

Zachary Brennan. "US to no longer distribute Eli Lilly's bamlanivimab alone due to coronavirus variants." Endpoints News, Mar. 25, 2021.

Shabir Madhi et al. "Efficacy of ChAdOx1 nCov-19 Vaccine against the B.1.351 Variant." *New England Journal of Medicine* 384 (2021): 1885–1898.

Robin McKie. "Pfizer and AstraZeneca 'highly effective' against India Covid variant." *The Guardian*, May 22, 2021.

Andreas Greinacher et al. "Thrombotic Thrombocytopenia after ChAdOx1 nCoV-19 Vaccination." *New England Journal of Medicine* 384 (2021): 2092–2101.

Nina Schultz et al. "Thrombosis and Thrombocytopenia after ChAdOx1 nCoV-19 Vaccination." *New England Journal of Medicine* 384 (2021): 2124–2130.

Eric Rubin, Lindsey Baden, and Stephen Morrissey. "Audio Interview: Efficacy of Current Covid-19 Vaccines against Variant Viruses." *New England Journal of Medicine* 384 (2021).

Eamon Dreisbach. "Pfizer and BioNTech say vaccine is 91% effective at 6months, protects against variants." Healio, Apr. 1, 2021.

Jackson Turner et al. "SARS-COV-2 mRNA vaccines induce persistent human germinal center responses." *Nature* 596 (2021): 109–113.

Apoorva Madavilli et al. "Three Studies, One Result: Vaccines Point the Way Out of the Pandemic." *New York Times*, Jun. 28, 2021.

Aylin Woodward. "Even more evidence shows vaccinated people are unlikely to transmit the coronavirus or get asymptomatic infections." *Business Insider*, Mar. 11, 2021.

Victoria Jane Hall et al. "Effectiveness of BNT162b2 mRNA Vaccine Against Infection and COVID-19 Vaccine Coverage in Healthcare Workers in England, Multicentre Prospective Cohort Study (the SIREN Study)." Preprints with *The Lancet*, Feb. 22, 2021.

Aaron Tande et al. "Impact of the Coronavirus Disease 2019 (COVID-19) Vaccine on Asymptomatic Infection Amongst Patients Undergoing Preprocedural COVID-19 Molecular Screening." *Clinical Infectious Diseases*, Mar. 10, 2021.

Testimony of Darragh O'Carroll and Derek Kawakami at the state senate COVID committee meeting, Dec. 9, 2020.

Dawn Gilbertson. "COVID-19 exposure on flights is more common than you think. The US doesn't share details, but Canada does." *USA Today*, Jan. 15, 2021.

County of Kaua'i. " COVID-19: Update, Jan. 11." Facebook video, 11:46, Jan. 11, 2021.

Allison Schaefers. "Gov. David Ige grants Kauai's request to opt out of pre-travel testing program." *Honolulu Star-Advertiser*, Nov. 27, 2020.

"Domestic Travel During the COVID-19 Pandemic." Centers for Disease Control and Prevention, Dec. 2, 2020.

F. DeWolfe Miller. *Surveillance of COVID-19 Infection in Pre-tested Travelers to Hawaii*. Nov. 30, 2020.

Amy Hou et al. "A Rapid Method to Evaluate Pre-Travel Programs for COVID-19: A Study in Hawaii." medRxiv, Mar. 8, 2021.

Notes from HICOVID meeting with Dr. Lorrin Pang, Mar. 9, 2021.
Personal correspondence with Chad Meyer, Jan. 11, 2021.

Yoohyun Jung. "What's Happening on Maui? COVID-19 Surge Is Largely Blamed On Holiday Gatherings." Civil Beat, Jan. 11, 2021.

Mahealani Richardson. "Waikiki clinic says it's seeing an increase in COVID-19 cases among travelers from LA." Hawaii News Now, Jan. 8, 2021.

Xianding Deng et al. "Transmission, infectivity, and antibody neutralization of an emerging SARS-CoV-2 variant in California carrying a L452R spike protein mutation." medRxiv, Mar. 9, 2021.

Kristen Consillio. "Health Department says highly transmissible COVID-19 variant present in Hawaii." *Honolulu Star-Advertiser*, Mar. 8, 2021.

Nikki Schenfeld. "Hawaii DOH detects more coronavirus variant cases." KHON2, Mar. 20, 2021.

Christie Wilson. "Health officials worried double-mutant COVID-19 strain could make its way to Hawaii." *Honolulu Star-Advertiser*, Apr. 10, 2021.

Hawaii DOH. "The Weekly Dose: Learn about COVID Variants in Hawaii." YouTube video, 17:52, Apr. 9, 2021.

Hawaii sequencing and variants of SARS-Cov-2. Department of Health, Jun. 10, 2021.

Allison Schaefers. "Residents' sentiment towards tourism has worsened." *Honolulu Star-Advertiser*, Dec. 21, 2020.

Dan Nakaso. "Hawaii residents support limits on tourism, survey finds." *Honolulu Star-Advertiser*, Jun. 2, 2021.

Managing Tourism in Hawai'i: A Survey of Resident Attitudes on Destination Management Issues. University of Hawai'i Public Policy Center, Jun. 2, 2021.

Stewart Yerton. "House Speaker: Changing Hawaii's Pre-Travel Testing Program 'Doesn't Serve The Public.'" Civil Beat, Nov. 23, 2020.

Noa Dagan et al. "BNT162b2 mRNA Covid-19 Vaccine in a Nationwide Mass Vaccination Setting." *New England Journal of Medicine 384* (2021): 1412–1423.

Shira Rubin. "After delays and ethics debates, Israel begins vaccinating 100,000 Palestinian day laborers." *Washington Post*, Mar. 8, 2021.

Pascale Bonnefoy and Ernesto Londono. "Despite Chile's Speedy Covid-19 Vaccination Drive, Cases Soar." *New York Times*, Mar. 30, 2021.

Eran Segal (@segal_eran). "Israel: covid-19 cases are much younger . . ." Twitter, Mar. 5, 2021, 5:21 a.m.

Eran Segal (@segal_eran). "Demographic split in Israel's COVID epidemic after vaccine roll-out." Twitter, Mar. 7, 2021, 5:38 a.m.

Nikki Schenfeld. "Hawaii DOH detects more coronavirus variant cases." KHON2, Mar. 20, 2021.

Gina Mangieri. "Rapid growth in Hawaii arrivals stresses Safe Travels coronavirus screening." KHON2, Mar. 23, 2021.

Nikki Schenfeld. "New study says testing similar to Safe Travels may detect nearly 90% of travelers with coronavirus." KHON2, Mar. 27, 2021.

Kehaulani Cerizo. "Maui study: More cases slipping through cracks of travel program." *Maui News*, Mar. 31, 2021.

Eleni Avendaño. "Kauai Tightens Restrictions To Slow Spike In COVID-19 Cases." Civil Beat, May 7, 2021.

Mathew Kiang et al. "Routine asymptomatic testing strategies for airline travel during the COVID-19 pandemic: a simulation study." *The Lancet Infectious Diseases* 21, no. 7 (2021): 929–938.

Apoorva Mandavilli. "A Riot Amid a Pandemic: Did the Virus, Too, Storm the Capitol?" *New York Times*, Jan. 7, 2021.

Neena Satija. "'I do regret being there': Simone Gold, noted hydroxychloroquine advocate, was inside the Capitol during the riot." *Washington Post*, Jan. 12, 2021.

"Second House member tests positive for COVID-19 after riot lockdown." WGN9, Jan. 12, 2021.

Louis Casiano. "Man in bearskin headdress in Capitol was booted from Navy over refusal of vaccine, report says." Fox News, Jan. 12, 2021.

Dan Nakaso. "Bill creating statewide Hawaii travel policy dies in House." *Honolulu Star-Advertiser*, Apr. 7, 2021.

Nina Wu. "Honolulu Mayor Rick Blangiardi won't change current tier system." *Honolulu Star-Advertiser*, Jan. 14, 2021.

Andrew Gomes. "No word on Oahu reopening tier changes as new COVID-19 cases rise." *Honolulu Star-Advertiser*, Apr. 3, 2021.

Samira Sami et al. "Community Transmission of SARS-CoV-2 Associated with a Local Bar Opening Event—Illinois, February 2021." *Morbidity and Mortality Weekly Report* 70, no. 14 (2021): 528–532.

Christina Jedra. "Despite Rising Cases, Blangiardi 'Dead Set Against' Return To Tier 2 For Honolulu." Civil Beat, Apr. 5, 2021.

Apoorva Mandavilli. "Reaching 'Herd Immunity' Is Unlikely in the U.S.,

Experts Now Believe." *New York Times*, May 3, 2021.

Chapter Fourteen

David Wallace-Wells. "How the West Lost COVID." *New York*, Mar. 15, 2021.

Ishaan Tharoor. "Brazil's rolling coronavirus disaster is a global problem." *Washington Post*, Mar. 16, 2021.

Colleen Barry. "Europe staggers as infectious variants power virus surge." Associated Press, Mar. 5, 2021.

Akilah Johnson. "Death in the prime of life: Covid-19 proves especially lethal to younger Latinos." *Washington Post*, Mar. 15, 2021.

Christopher Murray and Peter Piot. "The Potential Future of the COVID-19 Pandemic." *Journal of the American Medical Association* 325, no. 13 (2021): 1249–1250.

Lauren Frayer. "How India Went From A Ray Of Hope To A World Record For Most COVID Cases In A Day." National Public Radio, Apr. 22, 2021.

"Estimation of total mortality due to COVID-19." Institute for Health Metrics and Evaluation, May 13, 2021.

Fran Kritz. "Why 'Tight' Cultures May Fare Better Than 'Loose' Cultures In A Pandemic." National Public Radio, Feb. 23, 2021.

Kristen Consillio. "A year of COVID-19: Key leaders in Hawaii's pandemic response recall the challenges they faced." *Honolulu Star-Advertiser*, Feb. 28, 2021.

Christina Jedra. "COVID-19 Is Airborne. So Why Doesn't Hawaii Have Pandemic Air Quality Standards?" Civil Beat, Mar. 11, 2021.

Allison Schaefers. "Hawaii logs its best three days of tourist arrivals in a year." *Honolulu Star-Advertiser*, Mar. 16, 2021.

Anita Hofschneider. "Pacific Islanders, Including Hawaiians, Disproportionately Missing Out On Vaccines." Civil Beat, Mar. 16, 2021.

Dennis Fujimoto. "DOE announces 4th quarter schools schedules." *The Garden Island*, Mar. 9, 2021.

Caleb Jones. "Sheltered from virus, Kauai plans cautious return to tourism." Associated Press, Mar. 18, 2021.

Richard Read. "Kauai beat COVID-19, but now faces a new challenge: Rebuilding its economy." *Honolulu Star-Advertiser*, Jun. 2, 2021.

Paige McClanahan. "In Empty Amsterdam, Reconsidering Tourism." *New York Times*, Mar. 31, 2021.

Stewart Yerton. "Here's Why It's So Hard To Reshape Hawaii's Tourism Industry." Civil Beat, May 2, 2021.

Sophie Cocke. "Kauai sees spike in COVID-19 cases following relaxed travel restrictions." *Honolulu Star-Advertiser*, May 4, 2021.

"Hawaii COVID-19 Data" page, State of Hawaiʻi - Department of Health website.

Andrew Gomes. "No word on Oahu reopening tier changes as new COVID-19 cases rise." *Honolulu Star-Advertiser*, Apr. 3, 2021.

INDEX

ABOUT THE AUTHOR

Jonathan Dworkin is a clinical infectious diseases doctor based in Waimea, Hawai'i. A graduate of the humanities and medicine program at Mount Sinai School of Medicine in New York, Dr. Dworkin majored as an undergraduate in European literature, and he has always combined medicine with an interest in human rights. As a medical student, he traveled to the Kurdish region in northern Iraq and worked with the Kurdish government to document the sequelae of the chemical weapons attacks on Halabja. During that and subsequent visits, his work on medicine and the Kurds appeared online at the *Washington Monthly* and *Mother Jones*. During the pandemic, his writing was widely linked on social media, and in August 2020, the *Honolulu Star-Advertiser* published his piece on the state's faltering pandemic response.

Dr. Dworkin was the University of Hawai'i Resident Physician of the Year during his final year of training in 2009. He worked as the antimicrobial stewardship director, and as part of the infection control team, for the Queen's Healthcare System from 2015 to 2019. In 2018 he was named by Queen's as the Ke Kauka Po'okela Outstanding Physician of the Year. During the COVID-19 pandemic, he served as an advisor for the mayors of Honolulu and Hawai'i counties.

He currently resides on the Big Island of Hawai'i and practices infectious diseases at Queen's North Hawai'i in Waimea.